The United States Health Care System

COMBINING BUSINESS, HEALTH, AND DELIVERY

THIRD EDITION

Anne Austin, PhD, JD

Vice Chancellor of Research, Planning & Assessment
University of Arkansas
Community College at Batesville

Victoria Wetle, RN, EdD

Retired Program Chair
Health Services Management
Chemeketa Community College
Salem, Oregon

PEARSON

Boston   Columbus   Hoboken   Indianapolis   New York   San Francisco
Amsterdam   Cape Town   Dubai   London   Madrid   Milan   Munich   Paris   Montreal   Toronto
Delhi   Mexico City   São Paulo   Sydney   Hong Kong   Seoul   Singapore   Taipei   Tokyo

Publisher: Julie Levin Alexander
Publisher's Assistant: Regina Bruno
Acquisitions Editor: Marlene Pratt
Project Management, Team Lead: Cindy Zonneveld
Project Manager: Yagnesh Jani
Program Manager: Faye Gemmellaro
Program Management, Team Lead: Melissa Bashe
Editorial Assistant: Lauren Bonilla
Marketing Manager: Brittany Hammond
Senior Marketing Coordinator: Alicia Wozniak
Marketing Specialist: Michael Sirinides

Senior Operations Specialist: Mary Ann Gloriande
Digital Program Manager: Amy Peltier
Media Project Manager: Lorena Cerisano
Creative Director: Andrea Nix
Art Director: Maria Guglielmo Walsh
Cover Designer: Studio Montage
Cover Image: Shutterstock/Andrea Izzotti;
    Shutterstock/Tom Wang; Shutterstock/Levent Konuk
Composition: iEnergizer Aptara®, Ltd.
Printing and Binding: LSC Communications, Inc.
Cover Printer: LSC Communications, Inc.

Library of Congress Cataloging-in-Publication Data

Names: Austin, Anne, 1960- author. | Wetle, Victoria L., author.
Title: The United States health care system : combining business, health, and delivery/Anne Austin,
    PhD, JD, Vice Chancellor of Research, Planning & Assessment, University of Arkansas, Community
    College at Batesville, Victoria Wetle, RN, EdD Retired Program Chair, Health Services Management,
    Chemeketa Community College, Salem, Oregon.
Description: Third edition. | Boston : Pearson, 017. | Includes index.
Identifiers: LCCN 2015038599| ISBN 9780134297798 | ISBN 0134297792
Subjects: LCSH: Medical care—United States. | Medical economics—United States.
Classification: LCC RA395.A3 A955 2017 | DDC 362.10973—dc23 LC record available at http://lccn.loc.
gov/2015038599

ISBN 13: 978-0-13-429779-8
ISBN 10:   0-13-429779-2

Contents

Preface

Over the last several decades, literally hundreds of books have been written about health care. Some are general introductions to the field; some are focused on specific narrow issues. We decided to add our book, *The United States Health Care System: Combining Business, Health, and Delivery*, to meet what we believed was an unfulfilled need.

Of all those books, there didn't seem to be one specifically designed for community college students and lower-division four-year students enrolled in allied health programs. What these students needed was a book that introduced them to the breadth of the field of health care without overwhelming them with detail. And it had to be written in an engaging, easy-to-follow style.

In any introduction to a field of study, a choice must be made between breadth and depth of coverage. Health care is a complex subject; for example, whole books can and have been written solely on Medicare eligibility, to pick just one topic. As authors and community college instructors, we have chosen to err on the side of breadth. We have intentionally introduced many topics with sufficient detail to identify them and have eliminated nonessential details that merely confuse or bog down the beginning student. Our hope is that students will leave the class with a broad overview of health care and all its components, thus establishing the building blocks for further learning in subsequent classes and in their careers. We're delighted to offer a third edition that encompasses the many changes that have occurred both in health care and in the United States since the first edition went to production.

New to This Edition

- The Affordable Care Act (ACA) and its impact on the health care system and on individuals is well covered. The ACA has been integrated throughout the textbook and allows the students to assess the impact of this legislation on their careers and their personal lives.
- The Ayurvedic health care system is explored in Chapter 14. The author's personal experiences in Sri Lanka help make this an authentic examination.
- New Career Profiles have been added to all chapters, providing students with expanded information about employment opportunities in health care, with provider and non-provider options, including a full exploration of careers in insurance, pharmaceuticals, and more.
- Chapter 8, "Aging in America," has been rewritten to emphasize a broader and more positive focus on aging.
- The recent Ebola outbreak is covered in Chapter 10.

- Chapter 11 includes fresh material about the development of new drugs— and a description of just how a new drug is created.
- All tables and accompanying narrative throughout the book have been updated with the most recent data available through government and industry sources.

Unique Perspective

Our book is unique in that it combines a health perspective with a business perspective. Health care is a major component in the U.S. economy and provides many employment opportunities. Students are attracted to the field not only because of a desire to help people but also because their studies pay off with jobs.

The first author provides the business perspective; her background is in management and marketing. Her view of health care is as an industry and business, facing the same challenges of all businesses to maintain a competitive advantage in the marketplace. The second author provides the delivery systems perspective; her background is in nursing, health care administration, and bioethics. Her view of health care focuses on the delivery system and addresses the perpetual trade-offs among access, quality, and cost of services.

How This Text Is Organized

This book is organized around the pieces that make up health care. It addresses these questions: "What is this business called health care?" "How do we pay for health care?" "Who provides health care?" "Where and how is health care provided?" and "What else is included?" These questions are answered in the four parts of the book, in a total of 14 chapters, which permits the material to be presented in both quarter- and semester-long courses. The stand-alone nature of each part allows instructors to teach the material in the order that best suits their needs.

Part I introduces the world of health care. This section includes material on the size and scope of health care in the United States. The dual perspectives of business and delivery systems used in this text are presented as well as basic business and management concepts. The economic, government, and legal environments that impact health care are described. The payment process is presented as a framework for looking at health and money. The concepts of insurance and third-party payment are introduced, paving the way for subsequent discussion of managed care, Medicare, Medicaid, and other programs.

Part II introduces the people who provide care: those who the patient encounters first and those who work behind the scenes. Two chapters on clinical and non-clinical health care providers and professionals are included. We cover the roles of physicians and nurses in depth in one chapter and describe the roles of many other clinical and non-clinical providers in another.

Part III looks at where and how health care is delivered. It examines three health care delivery settings—the provider's office, clinics, and the hospital—to understand how primary and secondary care is delivered. This chapter describes the business organization, the roles played by managers and other business professionals, and the managerial decisions that are significant to these settings. Part III continues with chapter-length descriptions of long-term care, mental health, and public health. These are examined both as delivery systems and as specialty organizations.

Part IV expands the world of health care to include focused services and related industries. The industries of pharmaceuticals and medical technology are described to round out the student's understanding of the health care industry. Another chapter presents information about health care research and preventive care. Part IV goes on to discuss the important topics of cultural competency and ethical decision making. The text concludes with a chapter that provides an overview of the delivery systems in other countries as a counterpoint to the U.S. system that was the focus throughout the text.

How We Encourage Learning

This edition, as with the previous editions, was intentionally written in a straightforward, student-friendly style to facilitate comprehension by college students, who field-tested earlier versions. Based on our experience as instructors and the comments of students and reviewers, each chapter includes the following features to encourage student learning:

Learning Objectives

Each chapter begins with a preview of the material in a concise list of learning objectives. Students can use them to guide their reading and test their understanding of important points.

Profile

The text portion of the chapter begins with a real-life example that pertains to the topic of the chapter and is intended to increase students' interest in the material. One of the discussion questions in each chapter is related to the Profile scenario.

Career Profile

The third edition includes a new feature, the Career Profile. Every chapter includes a feature that discusses employment opportunities in the health care field or related industries (Chapters 5 and 6 already cover employment, and Chapter 14 contains an alternative discussion). Educational requirements, entry-level job duties, and salary levels are provided.

Exhibits

Each chapter includes exhibits. Diagrams or photos illustrate concepts or highlight the relationship between key points. Many aspects of health care are data based, and accompanying tables are presented to enhance students' understanding.

Glossaries

Like all fields of study, health care uses a specialized vocabulary that is often confusing and overwhelming to newcomers. To assist in learning vocabulary, key terms are boldfaced when they first appear in the text. Brief definitions are offered in the margin, and a complete glossary appears at the end of the book.

Chapter Summary and Questions

Each chapter closes with a summary of the key points that students should retain. Questions for Review test the students' comprehension of the chapter's learning objectives. In addition, Questions for Discussion allow students to expand their thinking beyond the facts presented in the chapter and provoke classroom discussion.

Chapter References and For Additional Information

Source materials are referenced in the text, and complete references are provided at the end of each chapter. The reference list allows students to explore topics of interest further and also models appropriate academic documentation for their own written work. Additional sources, including websites, are available for both faculty and student research.

Acknowledgments

We would like to thank Pearson for its continued support of this book.

Anne—All my thanks to Frank, Frances, and Kathryn for their ongoing love, support, and patience. Frank gets the credit for digging through company annual reports.

Vikki—As always I am grateful for the love, support, and encouragement of my husband, Myron, and for the joy given to me by Jonathan, Shannon, Clara, and Luna.

Reviewers

Andrew C. Rucks, MD, MBA
Adjunct Professor
American International College,
Springfield, MA

**Ashley Miller, MA, Public
Administration in Healthcare
Management**
Program Chair—Health Information
Management, Billing and Coding
Blue Cliff College, Alexandria, LA

**Janet S. Pandzik, MS Health
Education, CEHRS**
Project Manager—Healthcare
Management
Hallmark University, San Antonio, TX

**Jennifer Lame, MPH, RHIT,
AHIMA-Approved ICD-10-CM/
PCS Trainer**
Program Director—Health Information
Technology and Medical Coding
Southwest Wisconsin Technical
College, Fennimore, WI

**Nikki Bryant, MA, Adult and
Higher Education, BA Health
Services, Certified Pharmacy
Technician**
Associate Professor, Coordinator—
Pharmacy Technology
Ashland Community and Technical
College, Ashland, KY

**Patti Bundrant, BBA Management,
MS Healthcare Management**
Instructor—Healthcare Management
Career Point College, San Antonio, TX

Photo Credits

Ch.1 Fotolia.com/Stephanie Frey

Ch.2 Fotolia.com/ArtemSam

Ch.3 Courtesy of Wetle & Associates/Victoria Wetle

Ch.4 Fotolia.com/zimmytws

Ch.5 Fotolia.com/lenetsnikolai

Ch.6 Shutterstock.com/Tan Yan Song

Ch.7 Courtesy of Wetle & Associates/Victoria Wetle

Ch.8 Courtesy of Wetle & Associates/Victoria Wetle

Ch.9 Fotolia.com/gustavofrazo

Ch.10 Shutterstock.com/Tashatuvango; HHS/Medical Reserve Corps

Ch.11 Courtesy of Wetle & Associates/Victoria Wetle

Ch.12 Shutterstock.com/Ricardo Canino

Ch.13 Courtesy of Wetle & Associates/Victoria Wetle

Ch.14 Courtesy of Wetle & Associates/Victoria Wetle

The United States Health Care System

Combining Business, Health, and Delivery

1

Health and Health Care in America

An Introduction

Learning Objectives

After reading this chapter, you should be able to:

1. Define health and health care.
2. Compare the medical and wellness models of health.
3. Identify major demographic categories of the American population.
4. Describe key indicators of the health of the American population.
5. Describe the size and scope of the health care industry in the United States.
6. Describe recent health reform efforts.

Sally Meets Health Care Providers

Sally, a college student majoring in health sciences, woke up with a very sore throat and an earache. Because the college does not have an urgent clinic or any student health program, Sally called her primary care physician's office. After a phone assessment by the triage nurse, Sally was directed to come into the clinic for a throat culture because of the possibility of a streptococcal infection.

Sally raced to the clinic between classes, thinking it would only take a moment to get a throat swab. The receptionist had Sally fill out a patient record visit, used her computer to determine which phlebotomist had an opening, and asked her to take a seat. After a 30-minute wait, Sally was taken back to the laboratory area, had her throat swabbed, and was told to give the receptionist her cell phone number so they could contact her if she needed an urgent appointment.

She had missed one class but went back to school for her next class. A public health epidemiologist would have told her to stay home because she was exposing everyone in the class to her germs.

Sally got a message to call her physician. When she returned the call after class, Sally scheduled an appointment for that evening with a nurse practitioner. The nurse practitioner explained Sally had a streptococcal infection, which had to be treated with antibiotics; without treatment, there might be a danger of kidney complications. Sally went to a nearby pharmacy; her prescription was taken by a pharmacy technician and filled by a licensed pharmacist, who explained how to take the medication and what to do if certain side effects occurred. She took her medication as directed for the full 10 days. Sally was just fine at this point, but as predicted by our public health official, there were seven other cases of streptococcal throat infection in the class that term.

A simple throat swab generated a lot of activity that Sally never saw. Her chart was put together, notes written, and the laboratory results posted to the chart. Then a medical coder found the correct code to insert on the form that would be sent to Sally's insurance company. This involved analyzing the information on the chart—called abstracting—and then posting the code. At this point, the chart notes went to the medical biller, who actually put in the charges allowed and sent

Introduction

Discussions of health care bring to mind images of doctors and nurses, hospitals, and nursing homes. The nightly news gives us stories about the latest government initiative to improve our nation's health, the outcome of a big malpractice case, or the impact of rising costs on access to care. In this chapter, you will learn about health care in the United States. You'll explore demographic data that provide a picture of health in the American population. You'll also look at data such as how many health care workers are employed, who the major employers are, and how much is spent for health care services to understand the impact of health care on the economy. The latest efforts to reform health care are presented, raising questions that you'll revisit throughout the semester. Finally, the chapter concludes with a brief overview of the topics covered in this text.

the electronic form into the insurance company, where another medical coder verified the information, batched the file, and sent it on to the payer. The insurance company sent an electronic notification back to the physician's office verifying it paid the bill, the accounts receivable clerk posted the notice, and a record was also sent to Sally.

The state epidemiologist was given the report filled out by the nurse practitioner on an infectious disease and checked for other cases in the area. A public health specialist interviewed Sally and others in the class. The vector, or cause of the outbreak, was not Sally, but another student in a different class whose children all had come down with streptococcal throat infection from their grade school.

Meanwhile, Sally's ears had gotten worse, and she had an appointment with an otolaryngologist. After examining Sally, the otolaryngologist ordered more antibiotic followed by an audiometric examination to be done by an audiometric technologist 10 days after she finished her medication. The examination turned out to be within normal ranges, so no further treatment was necessary.

A few weeks later, Sally had a dental appointment for a routine check and cleaning: the dental hygienist did the preliminary exam, and then the dentist checked her X-rays and physically examined her mouth. The hygienist cleaned her teeth and prescribed a flossing routine. While she was in the office, Sally met a medical equipment salesperson who was demonstrating a new computer program that allowed the dental surgeon and orthodontist to take digital pictures rather than X-rays, which were then projected on a screen in the exam room, saving X-ray exposure for everyone.

During Christmas break, Sally had an appointment to check her eyes. At the ophthalmologist's office, the certified ophthalmology technician measured the refraction with a computer instead of the old-fashioned eye chart. The optometrist used this data to determine the strength of the glasses Sally would now need. She took this prescription to the optometrist, who fitted her with glasses.

Sally had to give the same medical and insurance information to each office. She looked forward to something she had heard about in class: a single electronic record that all her caregivers could access.

Health and Health Care in the United States

Any examination of health care needs to begin with an understanding of health and how health occurs in the population. You would think that defining health would be a simple matter, but it actually generates a great deal of controversy. Traditionally, health has been defined using a **medical model**. This model assumes that illness and disease require treatment; therefore, health care focuses on the diagnosis and treatment of disease. In the medical model, Western medicine is the answer to health.

In recent decades, there has been a shift of interest from illness to wellness. The **wellness model** of health care focuses on the prevention of disease and the maintenance of well-being. From the perspective of the wellness model, health

medical model
A viewpoint about health that focuses on the diagnosis and treatment of disease.

wellness model A viewpoint about health that focuses on the prevention of disease.

is defined as the optimal functioning of each human being in his or her mind, body, and spirit.

Which perspective you use to study health care will influence what data you select to examine whether a population exhibits health or not. It will also drive your decisions about how health should be achieved, including what resources should be allocated where.

A Snapshot of the American Population

A good place to begin the study of the American health care system is to look at some **demographic** data about the United States. Demographic data include innate personal characteristics of individuals, such as age, race, and gender. A key source of demographic data is the U.S. Census Bureau. The Census Bureau conducts a census every 10 years; the last census was in 2010. According to Census 2010, there were 309.3 million residents in the United States. The bureau collects additional data in the intervening years using the American Community Survey. According to data released in 2015, the population had grown to 316.1 million residents in 2013 (there is always a lag between when the data are collected and when they are available to the public). Table 1.1 illustrates some characteristics of these residents and the changes between 2000 and 2010.

Age, gender, and ethnicity alone do not tell the whole story. In later chapters, we consider the impact of culture on health and health care delivery decisions. As these population figures are further subdivided and trends are considered, a more detailed picture emerges. This data can be used to predict what might happen in the future.

Consider two trends that emerge from the demographic data about age and their impact on health care. First, Americans as a whole are living longer. Life expectancy is now 78.8 years from birth, the highest it has ever been. Men and

demographic The data from human populations that describe vital statistics, size, and distribution.

Table 1.1	*Demographic Characteristics of United States Residents*	
	2000	**2010**
Total population:	281.4 million	308.7 million
Age of population:		
Under 18	80.5 million (28.6%)	104.8 million (34.2%)
Age 18–64	165.9 million (58.9%)	163.6 million (52.9%)
Over 65	34.9 million (12.4%)	40.3 million (13.0%)
Gender of population:		
Male	138.1 million (49.1%)	151.8 million (49.2%)
Female	143.4 million (50.9%)	156.9 million (50.8%)
Ethnicity of population:		
White	211.5 million (75.1%)	223.5 million (72.4%)
Black	34.6 million (12.3%)	38.9 million (12.6%)
Hispanic	35.3 million (12.5%)	50.5 million (16.3%)

Source: U.S. Census Bureau, *Census 2010*.
Note: Numbers do not add to 100% because of rounding error and method of questioning.

women who reach age 65 can expect to live to ages 82.9 and 85.5, respectively (National Center for Health Statistics 2015). The second trend is the impact of the baby boomers. Record numbers of babies were born in the years 1946 to 1964. Between 2010 and 2030, the 76 million baby boomers will reach age 65.

Both of these trends impact health care. An aging population increases demand for home health care and geriatric care. As longevity increases, an interest in the quality of that life becomes a major factor. As a result, preventive health care, including well visits and diagnostic screenings, becomes more important. Individuals seek information on exercise, diet, and alternative treatments such as acupuncture and hypnosis.

Gender also impacts the demand for health care. Women have a need for reproductive health care in addition to their general health care. Women are more often single heads of households, and they more often live in poverty. Women tend to live longer than men. Because of these gender-related needs, women require more access to health care over their lifetime.

Census data also indicate that the United States has increased its ethnic diversity. The Census 2000 was the first time respondents could identify themselves as more than one race. Of those who reported themselves as "white" in 2010, 2 percent (about 7.5 million people) reported themselves as both "white" and one or more other races. The Hispanic population has more than doubled since 1990 and is younger than the total population. When demographic data are combined with health status data, you will see that different populations experience health and illness differently. In later chapters, you will explore the issues of how diverse populations can best be served.

How Healthy Are Americans?

Epidemiology is the study of the nature, cause, control, and determinants of the frequency of disease, disability, and death in human populations (Merrill and Timmreck 2006). In the United States, the **Centers for Disease Control and Prevention (CDC)** is responsible for collecting and interpreting volumes of health care statistics that present a picture of illness among Americans. Combined with census-type data, health statistics can be used to design strategies to either prevent illness or encourage wellness.

Based on responses to the *2014 National Health Interview Survey*, America's health is good. Over 65 percent of respondents rated their health as "very good" or "excellent." Level of education and family income are closely related to good health. College graduates were more than twice as likely to be in excellent health as people who have not graduated from high school. Those with incomes above $75,000 were also twice as likely to be in good health as those with incomes of $20,000. Since data collection began in 1997 there has been an increasing number of Americans who report that they did not receive health care due to its cost. The percentage peaked in 2009–2010 at almost 7 percent, but has decreased to 5.4 percent in 2014 (National Center for Health Statistics 2015).

In addition to surveying Americans, the CDC also collects and reviews all the health statistics that are required to be reported. For example, the cause of

epidemiology The study of the nature, cause, control, and determinants of the frequency of disease, disability, and death in human populations. Also the study of the history of a disease and its distribution throughout a society (public health).

Centers for Disease Control and Prevention (CDC) A group of federal governmental agencies responsible for collecting and interpreting health care statistics.

Table 1.2	*Leading Causes of Death 2012*
Total number of deaths	2,543,279
Heart disease	599,711
Cancer	582,623
Chronic lower respiratory diseases	143,489
Stroke	128,546
Accidents	127,792
Alzheimer's disease	83,637
Diabetes	73,932
Pneumonia/flu	50,636
Kidney disease	45,622
Suicide	40,600

Source: Xu, J. Q. et al. 2014.

death must be reported, which enables the CDC to track that outcome in the population. Table 1.2 reports the leading causes of death.

In the last century, huge strides have been made in terms of health outcomes. Over the last 30 years, the morbidity and mortality of the leading cause of disease has steadily declined by almost 50 percent. Healthier lifestyles account for much of that decrease. New vaccines have also improved health outcomes. Disease such as measles, mumps, chicken pox, whooping cough, tetanus, and diphtheria, which 30 years ago killed young children, have virtually been eradicated. However, widespread immunization policies must be continued to maintain such outcomes. Hospital discharges for children younger than 15 years have dropped over 50 percent in the last 30 years. In the last 10 years, new vaccines against hepatitis B, *Haemophilus influenzae*, and pneumonia have saved countless lives.

A road map of the preventive activities to improve American's health is presented in *Healthy People 2020*. The focus areas indicate major concerns of Congress, the **National Institutes of Health**, and the CDC. These focus areas are discussed in detail in a later chapter; however, access to health care remains one of the major goals of the country. The healthy outcomes are directly related to being able to get medical care when needed. National legislation signed in 2010 addressed some of the issues related to improving access.

National Institutes of Health (NIH) A group of federal governmental agencies responsible for the health of the nation.

The focus areas and patterns of disease in the population also direct research efforts. Research can be directed at cure, control, or prevention with the ultimate aim of minimizing the impact of disease on a population. Curative research gets most of the headlines, but prevention has the widest impact on the daily lives of the population.

The Health Care Industry

The health care needs of the American population are met by the health care industry. Used broadly, this term includes all the workers and business settings involved in health. The health care industry encompasses all types of workers who provide health care services directly or who provide support or business

Table 1.3	Economic Impact of Health Care Businesses		
	2007	**2012**	**% increase**
Number of establishments	784,626	830,813	5.9
Revenues	$1,668 million	$2,051 million	22.9
Annual payroll	$662.7 million	$804.4 million	21.4
Paid employees	16.8 million	18.6 million	10.7

Source: U.S. Census Bureau, *2012 Economic Census*.

services. The industry also includes all the different facilities and systems in which health care services are provided, such as physicians' offices, hospitals, long-term-care facilities, and laboratories. Health insurance providers, pharmaceutical companies, medical equipment and technology companies, and government agencies play important roles in the health care industry.

Health care is both one of the largest and one of the fastest-growing industries in the United States. In 2013, the United States spent $2.9 trillion on health expenditures, or 17.4 percent of the country's Gross Domestic Product (GDP). This figure equates to $9,255 per person. The majority of spending is for hospital care (32.1 percent) and physician and clinical services (20.1 percent). However, prescription drugs (9.3 percent) and nursing homes and continuing care facilities (5.3 percent) are also significant expenditures (CDC, *Health, United States, 2014*, Tables 102, 103). **GDP** (or **Gross Domestic Product**) is the dollar value of all the final goods and services produced by businesses within a country's borders. Table 1.3 presents some figures from the most recent *Economic Census* that indicate the economic impact of health care businesses. In addition to these establishments with paid employees, the nonemployer establishments grew 9.9 percent in this same period, to 1.9 million, with revenues of almost $60 million (U.S. Census Bureau, *2012 Economic Census*).

Gross Domestic Product (GDP) The dollar value of all the final goods and services produced by businesses within a country's borders.

Health Care Employment

The U.S. Department of Labor forecasts that half of the fastest-growing occupations between 2012 and 2022 will be in health services. For example, employment of home care aides, sonographers, occupational therapy assistants; and physical therapist aides is expected to increase by more than 40 percent by 2022; and medical assistants, physician assistants, physical therapy assistants, audiologists, dental hygienists, and medical secretaries by 33 to 38 percent. More information about specific clinical and non-clinical professions is provided in later chapters.

The health care industry will continue to expand. The Department of Labor has identified three reasons for the continuing growth in health care employment. First, as already discussed, the aging of the population increases demand for health services. Second, advances in medical technology, covered later in this text, have changed both the way patient care is delivered and the way health care businesses are managed. Finally, continued interest in managing costs will also impact employment.

Health Care Delivery Systems

The three major places of employment are hospitals, nursing and residential care facilities, and practitioners' offices. More than 4.8 million people are employed in hospitals, 3.3 million in nursing or residential care facilities, and about 6.8 million in practitioners' offices (Bureau of Labor Statistics 2014). However, these are not just places of employment, but complex systems that deliver various types of services to specific groups of patients. Each delivery system combines the business side and a service model to address not only the needs of the individual patient, but also the institutional and global nature of health. Some of the delivery systems discussed in this book are described next.

Long-term Care Long-term care (LTC) is and will continue to be one of the fastest-growing sectors of health care. The term *LTC* means providing health care services to an individual for more than 90 days. Although the majority of those needing LTC services are age 65 or older, individuals can be any age. A wide range of care facilities and professionals is involved in LTC. In 2012, more than 8 million people received paid services from approximately 58,000 long-term care service providers. A small portion of this care is provided in nursing homes (about 5 percent), but LTC also includes hospitals, assisted-living and community-based residential facilities, adult day care, respite care, hospice care, rehabilitation centers, mental health facilities, adult foster homes, and children's chronic care facilities. It is estimated that as many as 7 million people receive unpaid care from family and friends (Harris-Kojetin et al. 2013).

Mental Health The availability and quality of mental health services affect every family and employer in the United States. Most mental illness is a chronic lifetime disease that interferes with an individual's ability to participate fully in family life, work, and school. Data from the 2013 National Survey on Drug Use and Health indicates that nearly one out of every five adults, or about 18.5 percent of the adult population, has a mental illness. It is further estimated that only about half the people (adults and children) who have mental illness get adequate treatment. Part of this inadequacy is because of economic and insurance status, cultural barriers, and the stigma of mental illness, and part is related to the inadequacy of the system itself (Substance Abuse and Mental Health Services Administration 2014). Expenditures for mental health services exceeded $132 billion.

Public Health Public health can be seen in our everyday lives in things as simple as the crosswalk lines on a street that allow us to cross a roadway without getting hit by a car or the laws requiring construction workers to wear hard hats so that they are not injured by falling construction debris. It is also recognizable in state and nationwide campaigns to reduce smoking, heart disease, and cancer. Public health is seen every day by such activities such as nurses providing free immunizations to low-income children and police officers enforcing laws around seat belt and helmet use.

Health Care Policy

Health care policy attempts to address the issues of access, quality, and cost, as indicated in Figure 1.1. It is difficult to design a policy, however, that will accomplish more than two of these goals simultaneously. What typically happens is that legislators identify a problem and then focus legislation on a solution to that problem.

The most recent federal legislation, known as "the Affordable Care Act" or "Obamacare," attempted to address all three goals. As signed into law by President Obama in March 2010, the Patient Protection and Affordable Care Act was enacted to improve health care for Americans in three ways. First, the act expands access to care by increasing access to insurance. For example, individuals are required to have coverage, employers are required to provide coverage, and benefits under public programs such as Medicaid and CHIP were expanded. Second, the act mandates ways to control health care costs. The Medicare and Medicaid programs were significantly changed. Third, the law includes numerous specifically targeted mandates to improve the health care delivery system's performance and quality. Many of the provisions will be described in more detail later in this book.

Any time there are sweeping policy changes at the federal level, it takes time for these to take effect and for people to adjust. The Affordable Care Act has been amended twice, and certain provisions have been challenged in the U.S. Supreme Court. The 2016 election has the potential to trigger more changes.

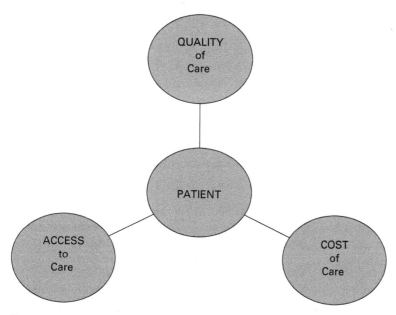

Figure 1.1   Policy Trade-Offs

How we pay for health care in the United States: Our system is a complicated process. Although the specifics are covered in later chapters, patients may pay directly or through insurance coverage. Patients who meet the eligibility requirements of age, income, military service, or some other status receive health care as a benefit. By mandating insurance coverage, the Affordable Care Act reduced the number of people who are uninsured and thus not receiving care at all.

The idea that something needs to be done to control the costs of health care is not new. A major shift in the health care industry over the last 25 years has been the shift to **managed care**. Managed care combines health care delivery with health care services. Two things are managed: one is the patient's utilization of services, and the other is the price paid for those services. The objective of managed care is to provide only those services that are necessary to contain costs. Although no one disagrees that health care has become increasingly more expensive, the shift to managed care as part of the effort to control costs has created considerable debate. A primary concern is that patients may not receive the care they really need.

managed care Describes the combination of payments for health care and delivery of services into one system.

Part of the focus on costs is because in the United States all industries operate in a market economy—they provide the goods and services that consumers indicate they want by paying for them. Business managers approach policy, or strategic decisions about the direction their business should take, from a **sustainable competitive advantage** approach. A business with a competitive advantage is able to maintain its position in the marketplace. Unless that advantage is sustainable, however, it will soon lose its position to its competitors.

What constitutes a sustainable competitive advantage varies from business to business and depends on the objectives the firm is trying to achieve. For example, a business could have an advantage because of cost: its product is low priced because its labor or materials don't cost it very much. This is why certain services are provided by a nurse practitioner instead of a physician. It could also have an advantage related to quality, either in its products or in its employees. Hospitals, for example, cultivate their reputation for providing the best care. A business could be competitive through speed: it's the first to offer a new product or service. Pharmaceutical companies try to be the first to market a patent-protected drug so that they will receive all the revenues from its sales.

sustainable competitive advantage Anything about a business that allows it to outperform other businesses and maintain its position over time.

Like health care policy makers, health care business managers must make trade-offs because all sources of advantage cannot occur simultaneously. And health care businesses must also try to meet the national policy objectives of quality, cost, and access.

Health care policy makers look to the major ethical theories of equality and justice for help in making health care allocation decisions. Most people will agree that there should be fairness and equality in the distribution of health care benefits across all parts of society. However, it will be clear as we study the health care system in the United States, and when we briefly consider health care systems in other countries, that fairness and equality are not easy to achieve. We will review some major ethical theories that provide a systematic way to allocate scarce and expensive resources.

This Book's Approach

This text presents an overview of health care in the United States, considering health care from two viewpoints. First, health care is a set of delivery systems that provides health care services to those who need them. At the same time, health care is a set of related businesses, all of which must operate as profitable entities. Figure 1.2 presents an overview of all the topics covered in this text.

The text begins by exploring how health care services are paid for. It is rare for patients to pay from their own pocket, so the systems and businesses that are in place to pay must be understood. The impact of the Affordable Care Act is discussed.

At the heart of health care is an encounter between a patient and a provider. This text describes the various health care providers and professionals the patient may encounter. The encounter takes place in various settings depending on what types of services the patient needs. These settings, ranging from the simplest office visit to the complexity of LTC, are presented next. Each setting is described both in terms of a delivery system and as a type of business.

Finally, other entities that influence health care are considered. In some texts, these are not considered to be part of the health care system because they do not deliver services directly to patients. They are included in this text because we believe that the business and policy decisions made by and about pharmaceutical companies and medical research and technology have an enormous impact on the patient. The U.S. system is compared with other systems in terms of form, costs, and outcomes.

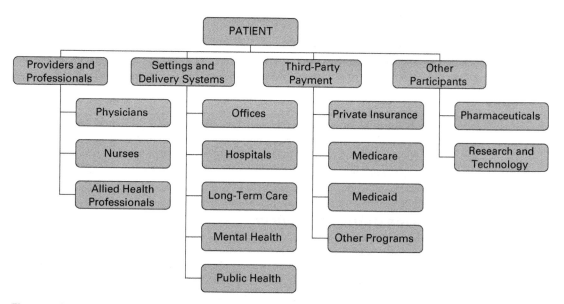

Figure 1.2   Organization of This Book

Career Profile: Statistician

Much of the information presented in this chapter is provided by government agencies such as the Census Bureau, the Centers for Disease Control and Prevention, and the Bureau of Labor, whose role is to collect and analyze data. All these agencies employ statisticians to perform this task.

A statistician's job might include designing survey forms such as the Census or the National Health Interview Survey. Statisticians decide who should respond to the survey and review the responses to ensure the data collected fairly represent the population of interest. Statisticians also collect data through interviews and experiments. Once the data have been collected, statisticians analyze the data and write reports of the results.

Biostatisticians apply statistical techniques to health-related fields such as public health and epidemiology. They also might work in the fields of biology, environmental studies, and agricultural research. The types of problems that biostatisticians research can vary widely from analyzing drug and alcohol use in certain populations to researching different treatments for a disease to evaluating new surgical techniques to assessing water quality in treatment plants.

The training for statisticians involves math and computer science classes. Biostatisticians also take classes in chemistry and life sciences. Most jobs require advanced degrees such as a master's or Ph.D. In addition to jobs with government agencies, employers also can include hospitals, university research groups, and pharmaceutical companies.

Summary

This chapter presents a picture of health and health care in the United States. Demographic data, such as age, gender, and ethnicity, were presented to understand some of the major characteristics of the American population. Health statistics, such as the major causes of death, were described, and the impact on the health needs and priorities of the country was discussed. The size and scope of the health care industry that meets these needs was presented. The criteria for making effective policy were discussed and compared to the criteria for effective decision making in business. Health care reform continues to have a major impact on the industry.

Questions for Review

1. Define health. What is the difference between the medical and wellness models of health?
2. List two of the leading causes of death in 2012.
3. List two health care occupations that are expected to grow by 2022.
4. Describe one provision in the Affordable Care Act.

Questions for Discussion

1. This chapter presented a list of the most common causes of death in the United States. How do these vary by demographic categories?
2. Why is health care such a large percentage of GDP? How does this compare to other segments of the economy, such as education, housing, or military spending?
3. Conduct a survey among your friends and family. What do they know about the Affordable Care Act? Is their opinion generally favorable? Why or why not?
4. How could the provisions in the Affordable Care Act improve Sally's access to health care (see the chapter profile)?

Chapter References

Bureau of Labor Statistics. 2014. *Industries at a glance: Healthcare and social assistance: NAICS 62.* Available at www.bls.gov/iag/tgs/iag62.htm.

Harris-Kojetin, L., M. Sengupta, E. Park-Lee, and R. Valverde. 2013. *Long-term care services in the United States: 2013 overview.* National Health Care Statistics Reports; no. 1. Hyattsville, MD: National Center for Health Statistics.

Merrill, M. R., and T. C. Timmreck. 2006. *An introduction to epidemiology.* 4th edition. Boston: Jones & Bartlett.

National Center for Health Statistics. 2015. *Health, United States, 2014: With special feature on adults aged 55–64.* Hyattsville, MD.

_____. 2015. *Selected estimates based on data from the January–September 2014 national health interview survey.* Hyattsville, MD. March 24.

Substance Abuse and Mental Health Services Administration, Center for Behavioral Health Statistics and Quality. 2014. *The NSDUH report: Substance use and mental health estimates from the 2013 national survey on drug use and health: Overview of findings.* Rockville, MD. Sept. 4.

U.S. Census Bureau. 2012. *Statistical abstract of the United States.*

_____. *2012 Economic Census, Industry Series Reports.*

_____. *2013 American Community Survey.*

Xu, J. Q., M. A. Kochanek, S. L. Murphy, and E. Arias. 2014. *Mortality in the United States, 2012.* NCHS data brief, no. 168. Hyattsville, MD: National Center for Health Statistics.

For Additional Information

Lee, R. H. 2014. *Economics for healthcare managers.* 3rd ed. Chicago: Health Administration Press.

Shi, L., and D. A. Singh. 2014. *Delivering health care in America: A systems approach.* 6th ed. Boston: Jones & Bartlett Learning.

White, K. R., and J. R. Griffith. 2010. *The well-managed healthcare organization.* 7th ed. Chicago: Health Administration Press.

The Business Side of Health Care

Learning Objectives

After reading this chapter, you should be able to:

1. Identify legal forms of business ownership.
2. Describe key business functions.
3. Identify the major components of the health care industry.
4. Describe the ways economic activity is defined and measured.
5. Identify key laws that influence the health care industry.
6. Describe how health care businesses can monitor and evaluate the external environment.

Competition Comes to Town

Dr. Anderson put down a copy of the industry newsletter and leaned back in her chair. Although her ophthalmology practice was doing well, the first discount eye care chain had just opened in town, and she was concerned about what impact it might have on her business.

Like most ophthalmologists, she had a solo practice. She employed an office manager and one technician. She also had a retail operation that sold frames and contact lenses. The glasses themselves were manufactured offsite. Two people were employed on the retail side.

Before the discount chain opened, her competition was the one other ophthalmologist and the three optometrists in town. The population of 14,000 had seemed to support them all comfortably. On the plus side, large portions of her patients were elderly: they needed the specialized care she gave, not just prescriptions for glasses. On the negative side, the town's largest employer, a manufacturing plant, was talking about layoffs, so those people would want the cheapest glasses they could get.

There weren't too many places she could cut expenses. One big expense was salaries, but all four employees were needed to take care of the patients. She had a long-term lease for the office and retail space at a good rate for the town. She had been considering some

new patient-tracking software and a new piece of equipment. She could delay both purchases, but both were intended to make the office more efficient and modernize eye care.

Maybe she could increase revenues. About 35 percent of her revenues came from the retail business; the other 65 percent was from patient visits. If she was open on Saturdays and in the evenings, she could see more patients. But she'd have to have extra help to cover the extra hours. She already gave a discount to a patient who had provided a referral, but maybe she could explore other ways to get more patients. At one meeting she'd attended, one doctor had given discounts for family members and for regular visits. She didn't know what the others charged for an office visit; maybe they needed to get together and discuss their fees.

On the retail side, maybe she needed to offer some less expensive frames in addition to the brands she already carried. Perhaps she could find a less expensive fabricator, although she was very pleased with the quality of the lenses they received. She wasn't sure if they had any customers from the other ophthalmologists; maybe she needed to advertise or offer second-pair discounts.

Tomorrow morning, Dr. Anderson decided, she'd meet with her employees and see what ideas they had for how to deal with this competitive threat.

Introduction

Businesses make decisions about the products they offer, the customers they try to attract, and how they organize and manage their employees and operations. As they develop plans and strategies, businesses must monitor and assess the potential impact of other businesses in their industry and changes in the external environment. Figure 2.1 presents these relationships visually.

In this chapter, you are introduced to basic business concepts, including organizational forms and key business functions. Key components of the health care

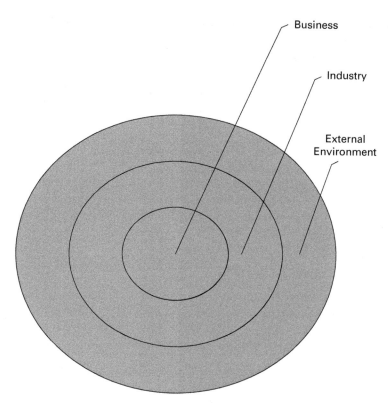

Business

Industry

External
Environment

Figure 2.1   Business and Its Environment

industry are presented. This chapter describes two external environments that impact the design and operation of health care businesses: economic and political–legal. These environments are the frame of reference in which business decisions are made. The chapter concludes with an example of one strategic tool businesses use to integrate their decision-making process with the external environment.

What Is Business?

Broadly defined, **business** involves providing a product or service to customers for a **profit**. When a business provides a product or service, it generates revenues by selling the product or service to customers. However, it costs the business something to create that product or service because the business has to pay for materials and labor and equipment. When these costs are subtracted from revenue, what is left is profit.

All businesses, regardless of industry type, must make a profit, or else they will be unable to remain in business. However, a distinction is made between a **for-profit** business and a **not-for-profit** business. In a for-profit business, such as pharmaceutical giant Abbott Laboratories, profit is the

business The activity of providing goods and services to customers for profit.

profit The amount left when a business subtracts its expenses from its revenues. If the amount is a negative number, it is a loss.

for-profit Making a profit is identified as the primary reason for the business to exist.

not-for-profit The primary reason for the business to exist is some reason other than profit.

primary reason for the business to exist. A not-for-profit business has something other than profit as its main objective. A not-for-profit hospital, for example, may focus on serving the poor in its community. The hospital will actually lose money on many of its poor patients, but as long as the hospital can generate enough revenue from operations or through donations to cover its expenses, that is okay.

If you look at a business that sells potato chips, it's easy to understand what the product is and who the customer is. In health care, those questions are a little tougher. Just what product or service does the industry provide? A physician's office could define its service as diagnosing illness or as preventing illness. Who exactly is the customer? The customer could be the patient, the individual who receives the service. It also could be the insurance company that pays for the service. How a business answers these questions helps the business organize and manage itself.

Forms of Business Ownership

In the United States, there are only three legal structures for operating a business: sole proprietorship, partnership, and corporation. Each has advantages and disadvantages, depending on the needs of the business. As you can see in Table 2.1, the forms vary in terms of ownership, personal liability, income taxation, and ease of formation.

Solo practices, most common among dentists and ophthalmologists like the chapter profile's Dr. Anderson, are typical examples of sole proprietorships in health care. In a **sole proprietorship**, one person owns the business. The owner makes all the decisions, takes all the risks, and reaps all the rewards. The *2012 Economic Census* shows almost 130,000 organizations as sole proprietorships.

A medical group practice is frequently organized as a partnership. In a **partnership**, two or more people work together to achieve the objectives of the business. Decision making, risks, and rewards are shared among the partners. There were approximately 68,000 partnerships in 2012.

sole proprietorship A legal form of business ownership that has only one owner.

partnership A legal form of business ownership that involves at least two people called partners.

Table 2.1	*Characteristics of Business Forms*		
	Sole Proprietorship	**Partnership**	**Corporation**
Ownership	One owner	At least two partners	Infinite
Legal Liability	Personally liable	Personally liable	Loss limited to initial investment
Taxation		Owner pays income tax on business's profits as part of individual income; entity is a pass-through	Corporation pays tax on its income; shareholder pays tax on dividends
Formation	Simple	More complex	Difficult

Nursing homes and hospitals are often owned as corporations. A **corporation** separates ownership and management. The shareholders own the business, but they give their right to make decisions to managers. Their risk is then limited to their investment, as is their right to receive part of the rewards. Corporations accounted for more than 167,000 health care businesses in 2012. S-corporations, a specialized form of the corporation for smaller business, accounted for another 320,000 businesses.

Although in a free enterprise system a business can choose which form of ownership best suits its needs, state law may determine the form of ownership for physicians and hospitals. These restrictions were enacted by legislators who wanted to promote public safety and quality of services. These forms are discussed in more detail in later chapters.

corporation A legal form of business ownership that can have many owners. The percentage of the business owned is determined by the number of shares held by the owner, also known as a shareholder.

Business Functions

Regardless of the business's legal form, providing products and services to its customers requires a number of activities. These are known as business functions and are presented in Figure 2.2.

Management is the broadest function because it involves people at all levels of the business. Management is the process of planning, organizing, directing, and controlling the business's resources to achieve the objectives of the business. In the planning part of the process, managers define their objectives and develop strategies and plans to achieve the objectives. In the organizing part, managers develop an organizational structure that helps the business operate efficiently. The organizational structure also indicates who is responsible for what. The directing part focuses on the business's human resources—how they can be motivated effectively. Finally, the control part of the process is a feedback loop. Managers must monitor to see if the business is meeting its goals and make adjustments if necessary.

management The business function of planning, organizing, directing, and controlling the business's resources.

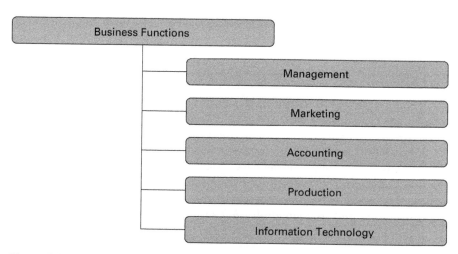

Figure 2.2   Business Functions

At the top of the organizational chart is the board of directors, the president or chief executive officer (CEO), and top management. These managers have responsibility for the whole organization. For example, the person in charge of a hospital is the CEO. Middle management refers to managers who have responsibility over a particular part of the business. The vice president of patient care, for example, is responsible for most of the nurses employed by the hospital. Line or supervisory management is responsible for a group of employees performing a specific task. An office manager supervises clerks, data processors, and receptionists. All the levels of management must work together.

marketing The business function that focuses on the exchange process between the business and its customers.

Marketing focuses on the exchange process between a business and its customers. Marketing develops a plan that includes the product, its price, promotion, and distribution to the consumer. Marketers do research to help them understand what products and services their customers want. A pharmaceutical company, for instance, develops a new product: a drug to control allergies. The company lets its customers know about the product by advertising on TV and in magazines. It sets a price for the product. Its sales representatives visit doctors to tell them about the benefits of the new drug and provide free samples to encourage physicians to prescribe it for their patients.

accounting The business function that tracks flows of payments into and out of a business.

Accounting keeps track of the money. Accountants track the flows of money into and out of a business. Money comes in when customers pay for the goods and services (called accounts receivable), and money goes out when the firm pays its employees and bills for raw materials and supplies (called accounts payable). Managers can use accounting data to make better decisions. For example, by analyzing cost data, a manager can decide whether the medical practice could save money by hiring an independent medical transcriptionist instead of using a full-time employee to do this job.

production The business function that designs and manages the process that manufactures the business's products.

Production refers to the process of physically creating the product or service. Managers analyze the process to see if they can improve efficiency without sacrificing quality. When manufacturing a product, managers improve productivity by considering factors such as how the machines are laid out. Similar issues are considered when analyzing services. A manager might look at the process of admitting a patient to the hospital to see where steps could be saved so that waiting time could be reduced.

information technology The business function that manages all the technology used to run the business and collects information for decision making.

Information technology (IT) refers to the use of technology to manage information. Primarily this involves computers and computer networks. Health care organizations collect huge amounts of data that they store, retrieve, and process. IT helps design the systems to do this as efficiently as possible. The move to electronic storage of patient data has created a new profession—health information management. However, patient health records are only one example of the data collected by health care providers. The business also has data about its own employees and other records concerning its vendors and suppliers. Legislation such as the **Health Insurance Portability and Accountability Act of 1996 (HIPAA)** impacted how this function is performed in health care businesses. The American Recovery and Reinvestment Act of 2009 created incentives for the use of electronic health records technology.

Health Insurance Portability and Accountability Act of 1996 (HIPAA) A federal law that mandates insurance portability and sets up procedures for electronic data exchange.

The Health Care Industry

As you learned in Chapter 1, the U.S. Census Bureau considers more than 830,000 businesses part of the health care industry. Under code 62 of the North American Industry Classification System (NAICS), the government tracks the activities of the sector of the economy it calls health and social assistance. The businesses in code 62 are divided into four categories: ambulatory health care services, hospitals, nursing and residential care facilities, and social assistance. Each category is further divided. Every 5 years, the Census Bureau tracks the economic activity by measuring number of employees, size of payroll, and revenues. Revenues are broken out by what types of products are being sold (U.S. Bureau of the Census 2012).

The Impact of the Economy

Businesses in the United States operate in a **market economy** (also called a private or free enterprise system). Competition is the central feature of a market economy. Anyone can open a business and offer whatever product he or she chooses. The business will succeed if it can provide a product that the market (customers) wants. The business must provide value—measured by the quality of the product and the level of customer satisfaction—to make itself different from its competitors. Dr. Anderson, the ophthalmologist described in the chapter profile, is facing the question of how to remain competitive.

market economy An economy in which many sellers compete for customers.

Some parts of the health care industry do not operate in a true market economy. In some geographic regions, there may be only one or two hospitals or only three dentists. A market where there are only a few sellers is called an **oligopoly**. If a pharmaceutical company holds a patent and sells the only drug for heartburn, then it is a **monopoly**. In markets where there is very little competition, sellers can raise prices and do not have to be as sensitive to their customers.

oligopoly An economy with only a few sellers.

monopoly An economy with only one seller. The one seller is able to set whatever price it chooses.

The allocation of resources in a market economy can be understood by understanding the demand and supply of goods. From the customers' side, the lower the price of a product falls, the more of it they are willing to buy. For example, if the price of cough syrup is $3.59, I might buy two bottles. If the price was $2.79, I might be willing to buy three bottles, and so on. This is the **demand** for the product.

From the producers' side, the higher the price goes, the more they are willing to produce for the market. At $2.79 per bottle, the manufacturer might be willing to produce one bottle; at $3.59, the manufacturer might be willing to produce two bottles. This is the supply for the product. As shown in Figure 2.3, the two sides meet at a point called the equilibrium price or the price at which the amount consumers demand and the amount that the producers supply are equal. In our example, the equilibrium price is $3.59.

demand The amount of a good a buyer is willing to purchase at a given price.

This basic economic model helps us understand the behavior of consumers and producers. The model can be used to understand why the price of generic drugs is less than brand-name drugs or why a nurse will change jobs to obtain a raise.

The health of the overall economy can be analyzed by studying data known as **economic indicators**. Among the key indicators that tell us how the economy

economic indicators Key measurements that provide information about the health of the economy.

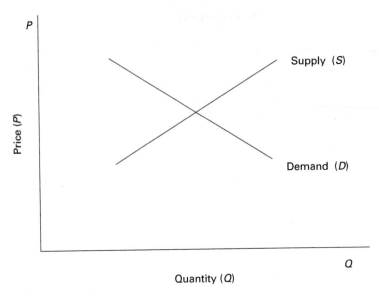

Figure 2.3 Supply and Demand

is doing are the interest rate, the inflation rate, and the unemployment rate. Studying changes in these indicators helps health care managers plan for the future (Lee 2014).

interest The amount, stated as a percentage, paid to borrow money.

Interest is the price paid when an individual or business borrows money. The price is quoted as an annual percentage rate. The lower the interest rate, the cheaper it is to borrow money. This encourages businesses and individuals to borrow, which allows them to spend more.

inflation An increase in the price level.

Inflation is an increase in the general price level, or average of prices at a given time. Inflation occurs when total spending in the economy increases in relation to the supply of goods, often during the expansion phase of the business cycle. Inflation has a variety of causes, such as a high demand for bank loans, heavy spending by the government, and a continuing demand for wage increases. Because prices tend to rise faster than incomes, consumers become afraid their savings will lose value as purchasing power declines. Often this leads consumers to spend their savings.

unemployment A lack of jobs in an economy for those willing and able to work.

Unemployment is the lack of jobs for those who are willing and able to work at the going wage rate. Although some unemployment is considered normal in an economy, economists become concerned when the number of unemployed rises above the normal level (called full employment). The health care sector generally has a lower unemployment rate than the overall economy.

business cycle Regular cycles of decline and growth in an economy over a time period.

The regular cycles of growth and decline, called the **business cycle**, pull together these economic pieces. There are four possible scenarios: prosperity, recession, depression, and recovery. Each is measured by the change in the GDP per quarter. Figure 2.4 presents the relationship between the key economic indicators and the stage of the business cycle.

In the prosperity phase of the business cycle, times are good—GDP is increasing, and the interest rates, inflation, and unemployment are all low.

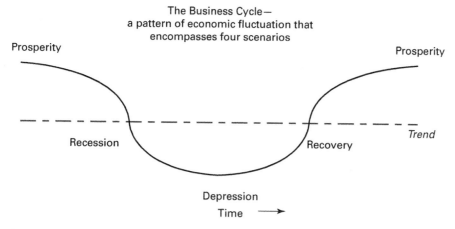

Figure 2.4 The Business Cycle

Because individuals have jobs, they have extra money in their pockets. This is money they can spend on items beyond necessities. For instance, an individual might decide to have elective surgery, get braces, or buy a pair of prescription sunglasses. Health care providers also spend money: they add additional employees, buy new equipment, and expand the office building. Businesses that are doing well might decide to add additional health care benefits for their employees, which in turn improves the health care provider's business.

In the recession phase, the economy slows down. Inflation and interest rates begin to increase. This causes businesses and individuals to spend less and to borrow less because these activities are more expensive. Individuals may only seek the health care services they must have. Businesses may lay off employees and cut health care benefits as they try to save money. Health care providers might also have to cut staff and postpone purchases of new equipment. All these strategies were seen during 2007–2010, when the United States was in a period of recession. The unemployment rate exceeded 10 percent in most areas of the country, and the number of uninsured increased.

If a recession persists, it is called a depression. Economic activity comes to a near standstill. Individuals buy only the necessities, and they may not be able to afford all of those. Unemployed individuals turn to the government for health care or do without.

The government may intervene in the free market economy to move the economy into the recovery phase. The government can lower interest rates and cut taxes to stimulate spending. In the recovery phase, things begin to improve. Businesses hire back employees, and businesses and individuals are able to purchase the items they need.

Economic cycles appear inevitable. The difficult part of a manager's job is to predict how often a cycle will occur and how long any of the phases will last. Like other businesses, the health care industry must monitor and assess economic conditions to make appropriate decisions.

The Role of Government

Even though the United States does not have a national health system, the government's involvement in health care is significant. Government actually plays three roles: as a provider of health care services, as a payer for services provided by others, and as a regulator of health care providers. The first two roles are discussed in other chapters of this book; government's role as a regulator is discussed here.

Government regulates health care by using the political process to make laws. The idea for a law can come from anywhere. Doctors and hospitals might want the level of Medicaid reimbursement increased. Older individuals on fixed incomes might want a law that sets prices for prescription drugs. A professional organization might want to change the licensure standards for its members. Each group would contact its legislator to make its ideas and needs known.

Industry representatives work with legislators to influence the political process. The American Medical Association and the American Hospital Association, as well as medical associations at the state level, lobby legislators to protect the interests of their membership.

Joint Commission (TJC) National organization that evaluates and accredits health care organizations.

Industries also create their own regulatory groups so that government will decide no additional regulation is needed. The **Joint Commission** (formerly JCAHO) is a case in point. TJC evaluates and accredits nearly 17,000 health care organizations in the United States to improve the quality and safety of health care services. Its standards are considered so good that TJC accreditation often substitutes for federal certification surveys for Medicare and Medicaid (www.jointcommission.org).

Traditionally the laws that the government uses to regulate health care have had two broad objectives. One objective has been to ensure fair competition in the marketplace. Another objective has been to protect the public.

antitrust An area of federal law that prohibits monopolization and other activities that lessen competition in the marketplace.

The **antitrust** laws are an example of how the government regulates competition. These laws are presented in Table 2.2. Basically, antitrust law prohibits businesses from taking actions that lessen competition. This can include mergers, attempts to create monopolies, and price fixing and price discrimination

Table 2.2	*Antitrust Laws*	
1890	Sherman Antitrust Act	Prohibits restraint of trade and monopolization
1914	Clayton Act	Restricts practices such as price discrimination, exclusive dealing, and tying contracts where the effect "may be to substantially lessen competition or tend to create a monopoly"
1914	Federal Trade Commission Act	Establishes Federal Trade Commission to investigate business practices that are unfair methods of competition
1936	Robinson–Patman Act	Prohibits price discrimination; prohibits selling at unreasonably low prices to eliminate competition

Table 2.3	*Consumer Protection Laws*	
1906	Pure Food and Drug Act	Established Food and Drug Administration; prohibits misbranding and adulteration of food and drugs
1938	Federal Food, Drug, and Cosmetic Act	FDA given authority to regulate cosmetics and therapeutic products
1962	Kefauver-Harris Drug Amendment	Manufacturers required to test safety and effectiveness of drugs; generic or common drug name must be on label
1983	Orphan Drug Act	Sets incentives and grants exclusive marketing rights to promote development of drugs for rare diseases
1984	Drug Price Competition	Shortens application process for approval of Patent Term Restoration Act for generic versions of certain drugs
1990	Americans with Disabilities Act	Protects rights of people with disabilities

(www.usdoj.gov/atr/). Health care organizations must make decisions within the boundaries of antitrust laws. For example, a hospital that limits the number of physicians admitted to its medical staff may be accused of conspiring to limit competition from other physicians and medical groups. A health maintenance organization (HMO) or participating provider option (PPO) might be accused of price fixing and price discrimination when it negotiates fees and contracts. Dr. Anderson, the profile's ophthalmologist, could be in violation if she discussed fees with other similar physicians in her region. Although potentially more efficient for the business, a merger of two hospitals or medical groups has the potential to lessen competition because patients would have fewer choices of health care providers.

Legislatures also pass laws that are expected to protect the public. Table 2.3 presents some examples of laws that are broadly related to the public's health. Some legislation designed to protect the public specifically regulates how health care providers must behave. Examples are presented in Table 2.4. Some legislation, like the Social Security Act of 1965 that created both Medicare and Medicaid, has been in existence for almost 40 years but continues to be important to health care businesses because of the influence reimbursement policies and amounts have on patients and providers alike. Some legislation, such as the Affordable Care Act, is relatively new, so its full impact cannot yet be determined.

An important piece of legislation that directly regulates health care is HIPAA, cited earlier. Although the law was passed in 1996, some provisions did not go into final effect until April 2003. Continuing debate about how the health care industry would comply with the law's provisions and whether the law would actually achieve its intent caused part of the delay. The legislation has five parts, or titles. Title I provides for insurance portability. Title II includes two major components. The first deals with fraud and abuse and reform of

Table 2.4	*Health Care Laws*	
1946	Hill-Burton Act	Also called the Hospital Survey and Construction Act; federal government funded construction of private facilities pursuant to a Certificate of Need; facility required to provide care to underserved populations; enforcement regulation passed in 1979
1965	Medicare/Medicaid	Part of the Social Security Act; Medicare provides health care insurance (including hospitalization) for elderly and patients with disabilities; Medicaid provides health care for the indigent
1989	"Stark I"	Amendment to the Social Security Act, which prohibits referrals to clinical lab service where provider has a financial interest
1993	"Stark II"	Expands Stark I to include referrals to "designated health services"
1996	HIPAA	Provides for health insurance portability and protects the privacy of health records
2009	ARRA	Special provisions to protect laid-off workers and to encourage electronic records technology
2010	Affordable Care Act	Patient Protection and Affordable Care Act; requires U.S. citizens to have health insurance. Expands government programs. Specifies insurers' ability to deny coverage and raise premiums

medical liability. The second mandates administrative simplification, which includes privacy and security provision for health data and requires electronic data interchange (EDI). Title III involves taxes; Title IV, the requirements for group health plans; and Title V, revenue offsets.

The American Recovery and Reinvestment Act of 2009 (ARRA) includes the "HITECH Act" (Health Information Technology for Economic and Clinical Health Act), which adds programs under Medicare and Medicaid related to electronic health records technology. In another section, ARRA provides temporary COBRA subsidies to recently laid-off workers to cover 65 percent of the insurance premium.

The Patient Protection and Affordable Care Act was signed into law by President Obama in March 2010, although some of the provisions did not take effect until 2014, and some aren't fully implemented until 2020. The legislation is often referred to it as "Obamacare" or the "Affordable Care Act." The primary purpose of the legislation was to expand access to insurance coverage through mandates, subsidies, and insurance exchanges; preliminary data indicate that the number of uninsured has decreased since 2010. The act provides mechanisms for uninsured individuals to obtain private insurance, mandates employers provide basic plans, and expands government programs such as Medicare and Medicaid. There are restrictions on insurance companies' ability to restrict access to health insurance or to charge excessive premiums for coverage. Some of the specifics are described in later chapters. The law also created a number of programs to improve the quality and effectiveness of health care as well as programs aimed at prevention. The Department of Health and Human Services has created a website to provide information about the Act, as well as a database for tracking insurance coverage.

Integrating Business and Its Environment

As you have seen, the state of the economy, as well as changes in federal and state laws, can dramatically affect a health care business. Although managers can't change the environment, they can change the business's activities to meet the demands of the environment. As part of the process of developing business plans and strategies, managers assess the environment. This involves collecting data to understand what the environment is like at the present moment. It also involves making predictions or forecasts of what the environment will be like in the future. Managers can use a number of techniques to integrate the business activity with what is occurring in the environment around it.

Many managers use a technique called **SWOT** analysis to determine where the business is in relation to its environment (Thompson and Strickland 2003). SWOT stands for *Strengths, Weaknesses, Opportunities,* and *Threats.* As illustrated in Figure 2.5, managers analyze the strengths and weaknesses of their business and try to identify opportunities and threats in the environment. Managers then try to match strengths with opportunities to plan for the future.

SWOT analysis
Amethod used by businesses to analyze the external environment.

Figure 2.5   SWOT Analysis

Career Profile: Networking and Security

Like all businesses, health care businesses rely on computers to do their work. Networking professionals perform the behind-the-scenes tasks to keep businesses operational. A computer network connects all the different computing devices using hardware and software so they can communicate. The connection can be wired (made with physical cables) or wireless. The computing devices include desktop computers, laptops or tablets, medical equipment, printers, and even the office phone system. The advantage of a networked system is the ability to share an Internet connection, peripherals, and files. The network administrator monitors the system to be sure everything is working and takes care of issues when it isn't. The administrator might need to install new computers or printers or update software. An increasingly critical task is maintaining proper network security.

To become a network administrator, a person learns about network operating systems and hardware such as routers and servers. Most classes involve both the theory and hands-on experience with devices. A person who wants to work in a health care setting should seek out internship opportunities in the field. In addition to obtaining an associate's or bachelor's degree, network administrators obtain industry certification such as the CCNA (Cisco Certified Network Administrator).

Computer viruses and malware continue to proliferate, and all networks are vulnerable to hackers. Network administrators are responsible for installing and maintaining software to protect against these threats. The network administrator also manages the credentials and passwords of everyone who has access to the network and routinely backs up the system. However, increased risk has created additional employment opportunities in the area of computer security. Cybercrime is defined as any type of crime that happens using a computer or website. Illegal network access, identity theft, fraud, and viruses are all forms of cybercrime. Computer security degrees are available from the associate's to master's level. The training focuses on how the crimes are committed and how they can be prevented and detected.

Summary

Health care is a business as well as a delivery system. Business involves providing a product or service to customers for a profit. Health care businesses must define what their product or service is and who their customers are. The business may be legally organized as a sole proprietorship, a partnership, or a corporation. Regardless of form, the business will perform the key business functions of management, marketing, accounting, production, and information technology. Two external environments impact the operation and design of health care businesses: economic and political-legal. These environments are the frame of reference in which health care businesses make decisions. SWOT analysis can be used to integrate the decision-making process with conditions in the external environment.

Questions for Review

1. Define partnership and corporation.
2. Define the four areas of management.
3. What items are included in a marketing plan?
4. Define interest, inflation, unemployment, and supply and demand.
5. What are the key provisions of the 2010 Patient Protection and Affordable Care Act?

Questions for Discussion

1. If a manager cannot control changes in the external environment, why should the manager be concerned about those changes?
2. Do some research. What are the current interest, inflation, and unemployment rates in your region? Have those rates been improving or declining?
3. What activities could a health care business begin during an economic decline to improve the profitability of the business? (Hint: Review the chapter profile and assess the probability of success of each of Dr. Anderson's ideas.)
4. Interview your employer or other health care businesses to discover what changes they have made in their procedures to be in compliance with HIPAA, ARRA, and the Affordable Care Act.
5. In addition to accreditation by TJC and federal laws, what other means exist to ensure patients receive quality health care?

Chapter References

Department of Justice, Antitrust Division (www.usdoj.gov/atr/).

The Joint Commission (www.jointcommission.org).

Lee, R. H. 2014. *Economics for healthcare managers.* 3rd ed. Chicago: Health Administration Press.

Thompson, A. A., and A. J. Strickland. 2003. *Strategic management.* 13th ed. New York: Irwin/McGraw-Hill.

U.S. Bureau of the Census. 2012. *Economic Census. Industry Series Reports. Health Care and Social Assistance.*

For Additional Information

Federal Trade Commission (www.ftc.gov).

Fremgen, B. F. 2011. *Medical law and ethics.* 4th ed. Upper Saddle River, NJ: Prentice Hall.

3

The Payment Process

Insurance and Third-Party Payers

Learning Objectives

After reading this chapter, you should be able to:

1. Describe what arrangements are covered by the term *health insurance*.
2. Identify who is and who is not insured and how much is spent for coverage.
3. Describe the interaction between the patient, the third-party payer, the employer, and the health care provider.
4. Define the basic terms in an insurance agreement.
5. Identify the major types of third-party payers.
6. Describe how third-party payers are regulated.

Insurance Reforms Under the Affordable Care Act

Implementation of the Affordable Care Act has made significant changes in how insurance companies do business. Insurance companies cannot deny coverage because an individual has a preexisting condition or cancel coverage if the individual becomes sick. Premiums cannot vary because of an individual's health status; they can only vary depending on the individual's age, geographic area, family size, and tobacco use. Lifetime limits on coverage were eliminated. Coverage was extended to children until they reached age 26. Preventive services were expanded and, in many instances, are now free.

To assist individuals in purchasing a plan, the Affordable Care Act requires states to set up a Marketplace (also called an Exchange). Some states have set up and are managing their own Marketplaces; in a larger number (34 in 2015), the federal government set up the Marketplace. Plans offered through the Marketplace, known as Qualified Health Plans (QHPs), must meet those requirements noted earlier and include 10 features: ambulatory patient services, emergency services, hospitalization, maternity and newborn care, mental health and substance use disorder services (including behavioral health treatment), prescription drugs, rehabilitative and habilitative services and devices, laboratory services, preventive and wellness services and chronic disease maintenance, and pediatric services, including oral and vision care. The idea is that all plans will be in one place, with clear language, so that purchasers can make a comparison between prices and benefits. Plans can still vary based on premiums, copays, and coinsurance. Some may include additional benefits, and many will only cover in-network providers. Tax credits are available to help individuals and families between 100 and 400 percent of the federal poverty level afford premiums; over 85 percent of enrollees in the first enrollment period qualified for the subsidies.

Considerable outreach was conducted to make individuals aware of the Marketplace. Assistance was provided to help individuals compare plans and to complete enrollment forms. Enrollment began on October 1, 2013, with coverage beginning on January 1, 2014. Unfortunately, there were early issues with the federal computer system that slowed people's ability to enroll. In July 2015 the Supreme Court ruled in *King v. Burwell* that tax credits were available to individuals who purchased insurance on the exchange created by the federal government. About 57 percent of those who enrolled were uninsured previously, which indicates that the Affordable Care Act is fulfilling its intention to increase and improve access to health care.

Sources: www.healthcare.gov; www.hrsa.gov; Majerol, Newkirk, and Garfield 2015.

Introduction

How services are to be paid for is one of the critical components of the health care industry. Most people use the term *health insurance* when they describe how they will pay for the services they have received. As you will learn in this chapter, health insurance covers a very wide range of payment arrangements. This chapter helps clarify what insurance really is, how individuals obtain coverage, and the categories of insurers and how they differ. A behind-the-scenes look at the process of paying for services is explored by following a claim from submission to payment.

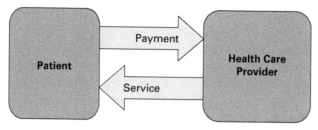

Figure 3.1   The Simple Payment Process

What Is Health Insurance?

Before health insurance became the primary method of payment, if you were sick you paid for health care services directly. You paid the doctor, you paid for a nurse, you paid the pharmacist for medicines, and so on. If you couldn't pay, you depended on charity or you did without.

As the cost of health care services increased, people began to develop creative ways to pay for those services. Plans that allowed prepayment of services, either on an individual basis or connected to an employer, have existed since the beginning of the 20th century. However, there was always the concern that you didn't know who would get sick or how sick they would be. Before health insurance, the family had to figure out how much to save for unexpected health care costs. But the family was never sure if they'd saved the right amount. A serious illness, then as now, could financially devastate a family.

Purchasing insurance is a way to handle that uncertainty and chance of financial loss. Insurance is the business of shifting the **risk of loss** from the individual to a third party. For example, if you own a house, there is some risk, or probability, that your house might catch fire and burn. If this loss occurs, like most of us, you will probably not be able to afford to replace the house and its contents.

risk of loss The probability that the insured-against event will occur.

This is where the insurance companies step in. You purchase insurance from them. If the house then burns, they replace the house. By purchasing insurance, you have shifted the risk of the possible loss to the insurance companies. The house burning is now their problem.

The insurance company is willing to take the risk because it can make money by doing so. Most people are obligated to purchase insurance to protect their homes. However, the chance is that only a few of those houses will burn. So the insurance company is predicting it will make a profit by taking in more money than it will have to pay out. The process is known as **risk pooling**.

Health insurance is a similar process of shifting the cost of illness from the sick person to the insurance company. Based on what it knows about your health and the probability that you will get sick, the insurance company charges you a price. As with the house example, it is predicting it will come out ahead because you'll stay healthy and not need the services it has agreed to pay for.

risk pooling The process of combining all the insureds into one group so the group's overall risk of loss is reduced.

The concept of shifting the risk of loss to another party is very straightforward. Health insurance gets complicated in the details.

Who Is Insured?

We protect our houses and vehicles from loss by purchasing our own casualty insurance. But only 5 percent of Americans under age 65 purchase private individual health care insurance. How do the other 95 percent pay for health care services?

For most Americans and their families, health insurance coverage is an employment benefit. Of Americans who are under age 65, 149 million have insurance as part of an employer-sponsored plan (Kaiser/Health Research and Education Trust [HRET] 2014). Fifty-five million are covered by Medicare; 70 million are covered by Medicaid (Medicaid, Medicare, and other government programs are covered in Chapter 4). This leaves 41 million people without health insurance. Some people have insurance coverage from more than one source.

Fifty-five percent of employers offer health care benefits, and 90 percent of workers are with firms that offer benefits. Among large employers (those with more than 200 employees), almost all offer health care benefits. In smaller companies, the number drops to about 44 percent of companies. Insurance is a benefit that attracts better-qualified employees and encourages them to remain with the company. Under the Affordable Care Act, companies must offer insurance that will pay for up to 60 percent of expenses, and the premium cannot exceed 9.5 percent of family income. Companies that do not comply will pay fees of up to $2,000 per employee (Majerol, Newkirk, and Garfield 2015).

Employees can opt not to participate in their employer's plan. Even in the companies that offer benefits, only about 80 percent of eligible employees choose to be covered (Kaiser/HRET 2014). Although some have coverage elsewhere (for example, through their spouse's employer), some are unable to afford the employee share of the premiums.

Health care is an expensive benefit for an employer to offer to its employees. In 2014, the average premium for single coverage was $6,025, and for family coverage it was $16,834. In the past year, premiums have risen about 3 percent (Kaiser/HRET 2014).

As premiums have increased, employers have passed the increases on to their employees. Although employees currently pay a similar percentage of the premium as they did a decade ago, the total amount in dollars has increased significantly—nearly 37 percent since 2009. The 2014 average contribution for single coverage was $1,081, and for family coverage the average was $4,823. In addition to contributing to premiums, employees share costs for office visits, prescriptions, and deductibles (Kaiser/HRET 2014). Actual amounts can vary considerably depending on the type of plan and the size of the employer.

Many insurance companies have realized that it is cheaper to provide services to people who aren't very sick or before they get sick. Most plans now cover common areas of preventive care, including prenatal care, annual visits to the gynecologist, and well-baby care. Some also include mental health care and prescription drug coverage.

There is a strong correlation between having insurance and being able to access the health care system. Most studies indicate that those with insurance are generally healthier than those without. The uninsured are twice as likely to postpone or go without care due to cost than those with insurance. If they do seek care, they are more likely to do without prescription drugs, again due to cost (Kaiser 2014).

About 16 percent of the adult American population under the age of 65 is uninsured, a number that has continued to decrease (Martinez and Cohen 2015). Most of the uninsured are from low-income families, and most are from families with at least one full-time worker (Kaiser 2014). Low-wage workers and blue-collar workers are less likely to have employer-sponsored health plans and less likely to participate if a plan is available (largely due to cost).

How Does "Insurance" Work?

When you compare the process in Figure 3.2 to the process in Figure 3.1, once the employer and the insurer are involved, the process of obtaining and paying for health care services becomes more complex than when the patient paid the provider directly. The insurance company, government agency, or managed care organization (MCO) is known as the third-party payer (sometimes just "payer") because it is the third part of the transaction between the patient and the service provider. This section of the chapter explores each relationship in the process.

The Patient/Employer–Third-Party Payer Relationship

When the individual patient or his employer considers which insurance company to do business with, it decides which company's plan offers the best combination of benefits at the most acceptable price. **Benefits**, or coverage, and price,

benefits The items that are covered under an insurance plan. Also referred to as coverage.

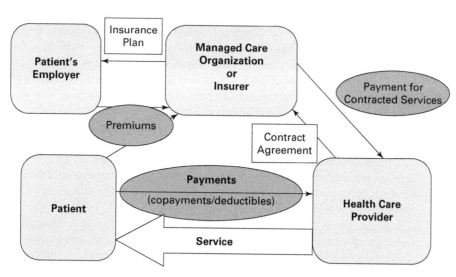

Figure 3.2 The Third-Party Payer Process

premium The price paid by the insured for insurance coverage.

or **premiums**, are a trade-off. The patient and the employer would like to obtain a long list of benefits—office visits, immunizations, hospital stays, mammograms, and so on—and would like to do so at a low price. But the more benefits that are covered in the plan, the more the benefits are going to cost.

The third-party payer will set a price for the benefit package. In addition to the benefits that will be included in the insurance plan, the price is determined by the number of people being insured and the general state of their health. As an outcome of risk pooling, the more people who are insured and the better their health, the more likely it is that the insurance company will not actually have to provide any of the benefits it has agreed to pay for. An **actuary** at the insurance company calculates this risk and helps the insurance company set a premium that will make the insurance company profitable.

actuary A professional who calculates insurance and annuity risks, premiums, and dividends.

policy The agreement, or contract, that describes all the terms and conditions of an insurance policy.

Once the employer has negotiated an agreement with the insurer, the employer can offer health care benefits to its employees. The employer is not limited to just one plan: it can negotiate with several insurers and managed care companies to provide employees with options. Larger firms are more likely to offer a choice of plans to their employees. The employer decides what portion of the premium it will pay on behalf of its employees and what portion, if any, the employee will pay for the coverage. If the workforce is unionized, this is often negotiated as part of the union contract.

insured The person who will receive benefits under the terms of an insurance policy.

The insurance plan is a legally binding contract known as a **policy**. If an individual purchases insurance directly, then he or she is the **insured**. If the employer is providing a plan to its employers, then the employer is actually the insured. The employer will have a time period, known as an **enrollment period**, when employees may decide to take advantage of the benefit being offered to them by the employers. If they take the benefit, they are known as **enrollees**.

enrollment period The time period during which people, usually employees, can sign up for or change their insurance coverage.

enrollees The employees who sign up for insurance coverage from the employer.

The Patient–Provider Relationship

Once the patient receives services from a provider, the payment process begins. Even though a patient "has insurance," the patient may have to make a number of out-of-pocket payments before or after the third-party payer pays for services.

deductible An amount specified in the insurance policy that must be paid by the insured before the insurance company will pay.

The first of these out-of-pocket payments is the **deductible**. A deductible is a dollar amount of services that must be paid by the patient or the person responsible for the bill as in the case of minors or dependents before the third party will begin to pay. Usually the higher the amount of the deductible, the lower the cost of the policy.

copayment (coinsurance) A payment made by the insured at the time services are received.

Most agreements now require a **copayment (coinsurance)** at the time that services are rendered. This means that the patient pays for a portion of the services up front. For example, that patient must pay $30 for an office visit to the primary care provider.

coordination of benefits If a service is covered under more than one policy, then the insurance companies determine which policy pays.

A patient may be insured under more than one policy. For example, a woman might have an individual policy through her employer and be covered under a family policy through her husband's employers. The policies will have a **coordination of benefits** clause that will determine which third party pays for services.

The Provider–Third-Party Payer Relationship

After the doctor or hospital has provided services, the provider now files a claim with the insurance company. A health insurance claim is simply a request for reimbursement for the services that have been provided. Accurate coding and billing are essential to this process.

Coding The initial stage of filing an insurance claim is the process of correctly coding what diagnoses, procedures, and services were provided to the patient. The provider selects the appropriate description of the service, and the coder assigns the number. The health care industry has moved toward standardizing the coding system by using two systems: ICD-10-CM and HCPCS. **ICD-10-CM** (the abbreviation for the *International Classification of Diseases, 10th Revision, Clinical Modification*) is used for physician office claims and reports diagnoses and reasons for the encounter. The other coding system is HCPCS (pronounced "hick picks"), which is the abbreviation for **Healthcare Common Procedure Coding System**. The HCPCS consists of two levels: **Current Procedural Terminology (CPT)** is for procedures and services performed by providers, and **national codes (HCPCS level II codes)** are for procedures, services, and supplies not found in CPT. (The third level, local codes, was phased out at the end of 2003.)

Billing Charges for services must be posted to client accounts. Claims are then transmitted to the third-party payer electronically. The claims are submitted on forms that are standardized for all payers. The payer replies with a transmittal notice and then begins to process the claim. An **explanation of benefits (EOB)** is sent to the patient to explain the results of the process. Payment is sent electronically to the provider. The amount of the payment will depend on what type of payment process is used by the payer, as described in the next section. If the payer does not completely reimburse the provider for that service, the provider may or may not be able to bill the patient for the difference.

Payment can be denied for a number of reasons. If there was an error in the process, then the provider can file an appeal. Other reasons for denial include incomplete documentation, noncovered benefits, termination of coverage, failure to obtain **preauthorization**, and out-of-network provider (Green and Rowell 2014).

Types of Third-Party Payers

Patients and providers alike use the term *insurance* to cover any and all third-party payment arrangements. Unfortunately, the term simply isn't comprehensive enough to cover all the variations of third-party payers that can occur. There are significant differences in the types of payers.

Indemnity Insurers

Indemnification is a legal term that means someone else takes the place of the person at risk. Indemnity insurance is the classic form of insurance. In a traditional

ICD-10-CM The abbreviation for the *International Classification of Diseases, 10th Revision, Clinical Modification*. This classification is used to code office visits to process an insurance claim.

Healthcare Common Procedure Coding System (HCPCS) A classification system used to code and process an insurance claim.

Current Procedural Terminology (CPT) A part of the HCPCS used to code procedures and services performed by providers.

national codes (HCPCS level II codes) The part of HCPCS used to code procedures and services not found in CPT.

explanation of benefits (EOB) A form sent to the patient that explains which claims were paid at what level.

preauthorization Many insurers require that certain procedures be authorized by the insurer before they are performed. Failure to obtain preauthorization may result in denial of the claim.

indemnity One party is exempted from incurred liabilities by the other party.

indemnity insurance agreement, the insurance carrier has agreed to indemnify, or pay for, the loss to the insured. With health insurance, the loss is the need to obtain health care services. In its purest form, once the patient has paid the provider for those services, the insurance company reimburses the patient (usually at a preset amount).

The insurance company may also reimburse the provider directly, usually on a fee-for-service basis. Payment is not made to the provider of services until covered services are used. Generally, indemnity insurance has no restrictions on the patient's choice of provider.

Self-Insurers

self-insured plan A plan where an employer pays for employees' health care.

third-party administrator (TPA) A company that manages the paperwork for an employer who establishes a self-insured plan.

Employee Retirement Income Security Act of 1974 (ERISA) Federal legislation that mandates how employer-funded benefit plans must be administered.

Many employers have shifted from traditional indemnity plans to self-insurance. From the employee's perspective, a self-insured plan seems no different than traditional insurance. In a **self-insured plan**, the employer assumes the risk of loss for medical costs instead of a commercial insurance company or a managed care organization. The employer must use its own revenues to pay for the health care costs of the employees as they arise. Often a **third-party administrator (TPA)** is hired by the employer to administer the health care benefits and process claims.

Self-insured plans are exempt from state insurance regulation. Instead, they are regulated by the **Employee Retirement Income Security Act of 1974 (ERISA)**. That statute provides rules for how employer-funded benefit plans, including health insurance, must be administered.

Blue Cross/Blue Shield

Most members of the public would be able to identify Blue Cross/Blue Shield as a health insurance company, but they probably would not be able to say what makes a Blue plan different from some other plan. Blue Cross was originally a group of teachers who paid Baylor University Hospital a small monthly sum in return for 21 days yearly of hospitalization. Many other hospitals adopted the idea. Blue Shield developed as a similar method to prepay physician expenses.

Today the Blue Cross and Blue Shield Association is a national federation of 36 local plans. In 2015, more than 106 million Americans were enrolled in some form of Blue plan (BlueCross BlueShield Association). What the plans have in common is the idea of prepaying medical expenses. Although most plans are nonprofit organizations, in 1996, some converted to for-profit status by establishing publicly traded subsidiaries. Individuals subscribe to a plan, so they are known as subscribers rather than policyholders. Local plans can develop HMOs and PPOs, and many serve as Medicare contractors.

usual, customary, and reasonable payment program (UCR) A method of reimbursing providers by examining what other providers are paid for that service.

Although the plans are a type of prepaid service, the subscriber is still responsible for deductibles, copayments, and any noncovered services. The typical way to reimburse providers is through a **usual, customary, and reasonable payment program (UCR)**. The usual fee is determined by what the provider normally charges for that service. The customary fee is based on the fee charged by similar providers within that geographic area. Finally, the reasonable fee considers any special circumstances of this particular incident. Determining the amount of payment can be a complicated process.

Managed Care Models

Thus far, the types of third-party payers described in this chapter are organizations whose primary business is insurance. These organizations do not deliver health care services; they only pay for the services.

Managed care describes both a system for paying health care providers and a system for delivering health care services. A managed care organization does both. Managed care has become the dominant mode of delivery because of its potential to reduce costs and increase efficiency. One of the key functions in a managed care model is **gatekeeping**. The patient can only access certain services from the primary care provider and can only obtain specialist and rehabilitative services if referred by the primary provider. This provides cost savings because only patients who are judged to need them have access to more expensive care.

Almost all workers covered by an employer plan are enrolled in managed care, up from 27 percent in 1988. Table 3.1 lists the largest managed care firms. As indicated by the revenue and enrollment figures, managed care is the dominant feature of the health insurance industry. In the past several years, the number of firms has declined as the industry has experienced extensive merger activity. A proposed merger by Anthem and Cigna is being reviewed by the Justice Department in 2015. Merger activity raises concerns about insurers' ability to pay claims as well as reduced competition that might lead to further premium increases.

managed care
Describes the combination of payments for health care and delivery of services into one system.

gatekeeping A process of restricting access to services.

Managed Care Structures

A number of organizational structures are classified as managed care, including health maintenance organizations (HMOs), preferred provider organizations (PPOs), and exclusive provider organizations (EPOs). Each is described in more detail in the following sections. Sometimes one company will offer several types

Table 3.1	*Largest Publicly Traded National Managed Care Firms, by Premium Revenue, 2014*	
Company	**Revenue**	**Total Enrollment**
United Health Group	$130.5 billion	29 million
Aetna	58.0 billion	23.5 million
Anthem	73.9 billion	37.5 million
Humana	48.5 billion	13.8 million
CIGNA	34.9 billion	14.5 million

Source: 2014 company reports.

Health Maintenance Act of 1973 Federal legislation that provided incentives for the formation of health maintenance organizations.

health maintenance organization (HMO) Employer prepays a flat fee to the HMO; employees receive services as they need them.

prepaid health plan (PHP) Refers to all types of health plans in which fixed payments are made before services are rendered.

capitation A payment method under which each patient is entitled to receive a set dollar amount of services in each time period.

staff model HMO Physicians are employees of the HMO and paid a salary.

prepaid group practice model Physicians are employees of an independent group that contracts with the health plan to provide services.

network HMO The HMO contracts with at least two group medical practices, described as "in network," to provide services.

independent practice association (IPA) model The IPA markets the health plan. Physicians contract with the IPA to treat members of the HMO.

of plans, which add to the confusion. In 2009, the majority of employees were enrolled in PPOs (58%), followed by HMOs (13%) and point-of-service (POS) plans (8%). Enrollment in high-deductible health plans with a savings option has grown considerably and now represents about 17 percent of covered workers; 27 percent of employers now offer this option (Kaiser/HRET 2014).

The **Health Maintenance Act of 1973** was a strong incentive for the growth of HMOs. The act gave the federal government the authority to provide financial incentives to new HMOs and required employers to offer HMOs as an alternative to indemnity insurance. An HMO could be formed under the new law if the organization could prove its ability to provide comprehensive health care. The act specified basic health services the HMO had to provide and supplemental services it could choose to provide. The HMO must document to the government its ongoing ability to provide services to continue as an HMO.

Health Maintenance Organizations **Health maintenance organizations (HMOs)** are a form of **prepaid health plan (PHP)**. Payments are made in advance of the services being provided. The **capitation** payment entitles the patient to a certain dollar amount of services over a time period, either monthly or yearly. Usually the payments are made by the employer, on behalf of its employees and their families. Whether the employee uses fewer services or more services, the employer has prepaid a flat fee to the HMO. If the employee uses fewer services, the provider keeps the difference. If the employee uses more services, the provider has to absorb that cost. This creates a financial incentive to provide fewer services to the patient, whereas the fee-for-service model such as Blue Cross provides an incentive for providers to give more services.

HMOs have evolved from the simplest prepaid models of the 1970s. There are currently several ways the providers of the services can be organized. In the **staff model HMO**, the physicians are employees of the HMO and compensated by the payment of a salary. This organizational structure is different from the traditional structure for a primary care provider (described elsewhere in the text). In the **prepaid group practice model**, the physicians are employees of an independent group that contracts with the health plan to provide services. In a **network HMO**, the HMO contracts with at least two group practices to provide services. Finally, in the **independent practice association (IPA) model**, physicians contract independently with the IPA to treat the members of the HMO. The physician is reimbursed on a **fee-for-service** or capitation basis as treatment is provided. The IPA is basically the organization that markets the health plan.

Prepaid health plans are attractive to employers because they know in advance what the cost of providing health care will be. They are also attractive to the service provider because the number of patients is fixed and a certain revenue level is guaranteed. Service providers are given financial incentives to control costs by a withholding amount. A percentage of the payment from the employer is withheld until the end of the year. If services have been overutilized, then the HMO keeps that money. But if services are under the stated utilization rate, then the withheld amount is paid to the provider.

Preferred Provider Organizations A **preferred provider organization (PPO)** is a delivery network. The PPO does not receive premiums or assume financial risk. Instead it acts as the go-between, negotiating and managing contracts on the part of providers. The patient may choose his or her physician or hospital. If the patient chooses to use a preferred provider, services are provided at a lower cost. If the patient chooses a provider who is not preferred, those services are provided at a higher rate. The patient gets more benefits by using the preferred provider.

Exclusive Provider Organizations **Exclusive provider organizations (EPOs)** have features that are similar to both HMOs and PPOs. A patient must select his or her care providers from those in the network. This is what makes the organization exclusive. If the patient chooses to go outside the network, then those services are not covered by the EPO. Unlike HMOs and PPOs, EPOs are regulated by state insurance law.

Regulation of Third-Party Payers

Insurance is a regulated industry. State governments have the authority to regulate the insurance companies that operate with their boundaries and sell products to their citizens. The agency charged with regulatory authority is usually called the insurance commission. The agency regulates all insurers, not just those who sell health insurance products.

Insurance companies must be licensed. As part of the process of issuing a license, the state reviews the company's financial health, its business practices, the policy forms it uses, whom it insures, and the premiums it charges. The intent of this review is to make sure that the policyholders receive the coverage they were promised and that they paid for.

Because HMOs and other managed care organizations are not technically insurance companies but are classified as health care providers, they are regulated differently. Most states regulate HMOs by separate statute. However, the intent is similar to the regulation of insurance. In addition, HMO statutes also set standards for the provider side of the HMO. Thus, they set out processes for consumer complaints, quality review, and utilization review.

Many states have added additional consumer protection statutes. All 50 states now mandate breast cancer screening as a benefit that must be provided. Twenty-two states insist on mental health parity. External review of health plan decisions is required in 44 states.

At the federal level, the Health Insurance Portability and Accountability Act (HIPAA) regulates portability, access, and mandated benefits. Congress also recognized the close relationship between employment and coverage by passing COBRA (Consolidated Omnibus Budget Reconciliation Act). COBRA provides that the employee may continue to be insured through the employer's plan even after the employment relationship has terminated. The catch is that now the employee picks up the total cost. Because obtaining coverage as an individual is

fee-for-service A method of reimbursement that pre-sets the fee that will be paid for the service that is provided.

preferred provider organization (PPO) A delivery network that manages and negotiates contracts on behalf of the providers, who provide services at lower cost.

exclusive provider organizations (EPOs) Delivery networks in which patients must use the services of those providers.

prohibitively expensive, COBRA provides a way of staying insured. During 2009–2010, there was a temporary expansion of COBRA as a mechanism to maintain insurance during a recessionary period.

The chapter profile provides an overview of the Affordable Care Act and the requirements it has placed on insurers.

Career Profile: Careers in Insurance

This chapter has focused on health insurance and how that system works. The other types of insurance are life insurance and property and casualty insurance. Taken as a whole, the insurance industry employs about 2.5 million people in a variety of positions. Your interactions have probably been with an agent or broker. Agents and brokers have to have good people and communication skills so they can inform clients about the insurance products they sell. Although there is no required degree, coursework in business and public speaking helps. Agents must be licensed by their state. Most agents work on commission, so if you're good at selling, you can make an excellent living. Claims adjusters and examiners also do not need a degree for entry-level positions, although earning a bachelor's can help with advancement. Adjusters and examiners review the claims made by policyholders and determine if the claims should be paid. Examiners often work on contract for an hourly wage. Actuaries and underwriters perform the highly technical work of determining the level of risk connected to a particular situation and how to price a policy. Both areas require excellent skills in math and statistics. Most underwriters have at least a bachelor's degree in finance, and actuaries study in actuarial science programs and must sit for several exams. Like any business, insurance companies also require people in all of the business functions that were described in Chapter 2—management, marketing, accounting, and IT.

Summary

Health insurance is a way to shift the possibility of financial loss caused by illness from the patient to the insurance company. Most Americans obtain health insurance through their employer as a benefit. The cost of the premiums is usually shared between the employer and the employee. Rising premiums are an ever-present concern to both employers and patients. Some costs have already been passed to the employee, such as higher deductibles and copayments for office visits and prescription drugs. Although all forms of third-party payment are called insurance by the public, only a few are traditional indemnity insurance plans. Various prepaid options also exist. Managed care organizations combine paying for and providing services in one business. These organizations can be structured as HMOs (health maintenance organizations), PPOs (preferred provider organizations), and EPOs (exclusive provider organizations). Whatever the form, health insurance is regulated at both the state and the federal levels.

Questions for Review

1. What is risk of loss? How does insurance address this problem?
2. Provide a profile of insurance coverage for Americans.
3. Define the following terms: *policy, deductible, coinsurance, premium, claim.*
4. Define self-insured plan, HMO, PPO, EPO.
5. Who licenses insurance companies?

Questions for Discussion

1. Why is insurance so complicated? Can the process be simplified?
2. Review a health insurance policy. What's covered? What's not covered? Do you understand the terms and conditions of the policy?
3. Refer to the profile at the beginning of the chapter. How is the Marketplace set up in your state?
4. Does the requirement of referral from the primary care physician keep costs down?
5. Some people feel that quality of care is compromised in the third-party payment system. What do you think?
6. How has the Affordable Care Act impacted you, your family, and/or your employer?

Chapter References

BlueCross BlueShield Association (www.bcbs.com/about-the-association/).

Green, M. A., and J. C. Rowell. 2014. *Understanding health insurance: A guide to billing and reimbursement.* 12th ed. New York: Cengage Learning.

The Kaiser Commission on Medicaid and the Uninsured. October 2014. *Key facts about the uninsured population.* Washington, DC: Author.

Kaiser Family Foundation and Health Research and Educational Trust (HRET). 2014. *Employer health benefits. 2014 Summary of findings.* Washington, DC: Author.

Majerol, M., V. Newkirk, and R. Garfield. January 2015. *The uninsured: A primer. Key facts about health insurance and the uninsured in America.* Washington, DC: The Kaiser Commission on Medicaid and the Uninsured.

Martinez, M., and R. Cohen. March 2015. *Health insurance coverage: Early release of estimates from the National Health Interview Survey, January–September 2014.* Washington, DC: National Center for Health Statistics.

U.S. Census Bureau. *Statistical abstract of the United States: 2007.* Washington, DC: U.S. Government Printing Office.

For Additional Information

Kongstvedt, P. R. 2015. *Health insurance and managed care: What they are and how they work.* 4th ed. Burlington, MA: Jones and Bartlett Learning.

Medicare E

GROUP
HEALTH PL
(SSN or ID

(VA File #)

3. PATIENT'S BIR
MM   DD

s SSN)

le Initial)

6. PATIENT R

4

The Payment Process

Government Payment Programs

Learning Objectives

After reading this chapter, you should be able to:

1. Identify when a person is eligible for Medicare and what benefits are covered.

2. Describe how providers are reimbursed for Medicare services.

3. Identify when a person is eligible for Medicaid and what benefits are covered.

4. Describe how providers are reimbursed for Medicaid services.

5. Define CHIP and identify who is eligible under this program.

6. Describe how fraud and abuse occur and what penalties are imposed.

7. Describe health insurance programs for government workers and military personnel.

8. Identify when a person is eligible for workers' compensation.

9. Describe how workers' compensation is funded.

The Affordable Care Act Expands Medicaid

As you will see in more detail later in this chapter, for over 50 years Medicaid has been the primary source of health coverage for the poor. Acting with the intention to reduce the number of Americans who are uninsured, one of the key provisions in the Affordable Care Act substantially expanded the eligibility requirements of Medicaid. States are permitted to expand Medicaid services to nonelderly adults with incomes up to 138 percent of the Federal Poverty Level (FPL). The law intended for this expansion to be mandatory for all states. However, a 2012 Supreme Court decision made the expansion optional. As of 2015, 29 states have adopted the expansion, 6 are discussing it, and 16 are not currently expanding (there is no deadline for a final decision). The federal government provided 100 percent of the funds to cover the newly insured until 2016; after that the government pay 90 percent. As a result of this expansion, more than 10 million people enrolled in Medicaid. Some of the biggest gains came in the poorer states, such as Arkansas and Kentucky, that historically have experienced high rates of uninsured. Although Medicaid expenditures have increased (as expected), states should see decreases in spending for uncompensated care. There is also potential for job growth and other impacts. As you might expect, a great deal of attention is focused on how the changes are actually working out on a state-by-state basis.

In addition to eligibility expansion, the Affordable Care Act has changes that are applicable in all states. States must modernize and simplify their enrollment processes and simplify how they calculate income. They also must create an enrollment system that coordinates eligibility for Medicaid, CHIP, and the Marketplace. To stimulate innovation, there are provisions for preventive and primary care through accountable care organizations (ACOs) and patient-centered medical homes. There are incentives to shift how long-term care is delivered, and most states have adopted at least one of the six proposed options.

Source: Paradise, J. *Medicaid moving forward*. March 2015. The Kaiser Commission on Medicaid and the Uninsured.

Introduction

In addition to payments for services through the private health insurance plans you learned about in Chapter 3, health care costs can be paid by several government programs. The two dominant programs are Medicare and Medicaid. Medicare provides health care services for the elderly; Medicaid provides services for the poor of all ages. In addition, there are special programs for children, government workers, and military personnel. Workers' compensation pays for work-related injuries. Although the government administers workers' compensation, it is funded by payments by employers. In this chapter, you will learn the details of each of these programs and consider the issues facing federal and state government as health care costs continue to rise.

Medicare

The **Medicare** program was created in 1965 as part of the Social Security Act. At this time, it is administered by the **Centers for Medicare & Medicaid Services (CMS)**, formerly known as the Health Care Financing Administration (HCFA). CMS is part of the Department of Health and Human Services (HHS). Because Medicare is a purely federal program, the federal government establishes the rules for who is eligible, what benefits are covered, and how health care providers are reimbursed. Medicare is financed by payroll taxes, government revenues, and premiums paid by the beneficiaries.

Not only have overall health expenditures grown dramatically since the 1960s, but also Medicare's share has more than quadrupled. In 2013, national health expenditures were $2.91 trillion; Medicare accounted for 20 percent of these. In 1966, the number was only 4.1 percent of $45.1 billion (Centers for Medicare & Medicaid Services 2015).

Medicare A federal program that pays health care costs for the elderly, the permanently disabled, and those with end-stage renal disease.

Centers for Medicare & Medicaid Services (CMS) The federal agency that administers the Medicare and Medicaid programs; previously known as the Health Care Financing Administration (HCFA).

Eligibility

An individual qualifies for Medicare in three ways: if he or she is over 65 and is eligible for Social Security retirement benefits, is permanently disabled, or has end-stage renal disease. Eighty-four percent of those enrolled in Medicare are eligible because of their age; almost 12 percent of the total U.S. population is over age 65. Table 4.1 provides information about the number of people enrolled in the Medicare program.

Covered Benefits

Similar to a private health insurance plan, Medicare benefits include hospital care and physician services (www.medicare.gov). **Part A** of Medicare is hospital insurance. Part A covers inpatient hospital services, critical access hospitals, skilled nursing facilities (not custodial or long term), limited and medically necessary home health care services, and hospice. An individual does not have to pay premiums to have Part A coverage if he or she paid Medicare taxes while working. Like other insurance, Medicare requires a deductible and coinsurance or copayment. The deductible varies depending on the service and the enrollee's plan.

Medicare Part A This part of the Medicare program pays for inpatient hospital services, critical access hospitals, and skilled nursing facilities.

Table 4.1	Medicare Enrollees (in millions of people)			
	1980	**1990**	**2000**	**2015**
Total	28.5	34.2	39.6	55.2
Over 65	25.5	30.9	34.2	46.1
Disabled	3.0	3.3	5.4	9.1

Source: U.S. Census Bureau, *Statistical Abstract of the United States: 2010,* Table 139; *CMS Fast Facts* March 2015.

Medicare Part B This part of the Medicare program pays for physician services, outpatient hospital care, and some services and supplies.

Medicare Part C This part of the Medicare program is an additional insurance plan intended to cover the gaps in Part A and Part B coverage.

Medicare Prescription Drug, Improvement, and Modernization Act of 2003 The most recent modification of the federal legislation. In particular, it added coverage for prescription drugs.

Medicare Part D This part of the Medicare program covers prescription drugs.

Medicare Advantage A revision of the Medicare+Choice offered under Part C of Medicare.

Part B covers physician services, outpatient hospital care, and some services and supplies. An individual who chooses to have Part B coverage pays monthly premiums. In 2015, the premium was $104.90 per month if the individual's income was less than $85,000. When care is received, the individual pays the deductible and a copayment for the service. In 2015, the deductible was $147.

Except for a limited time period following inpatient hospital care, Medicare does not cover long-term nursing care or home health care, both important issues for the elderly. Table 4.2 presents data on Medicare expenditures and persons served.

A number of modifications have been made to the Medicare program in an attempt to control costs. As part of the Balanced Budget Act of 1997, **Part C**, known as Medicare+Choice, was added to Medicare. Medicare+Choice offered individuals a variety of managed care–type options to provide the services covered under Parts A and B. The **Medicare Prescription Drug, Improvement, and Modernization Act of 2003 (MMA)** added new coverage for prescriptions and preventive care (**Medicare Part D**), replaced Medicare+Choice with **Medicare Advantage** and added new Medigap plans, and made changes to fee-for-service payments. The 2009 American Recovery and Reinvestment Act added additional services such as cardiac rehab and HIV screening to enhance preventive care and wellness. The Affordable Care Act made numerous specific changes, including closing the coverage gap in Medicare Part D and improving coverage of prevention benefits.

More than 35 million people are enrolled in Medicare Part D. There is no additional premium for this coverage until your income reaches $85,000. Currently, the annual deductible is $320. Medicare pays about 75 percent until expenses reach $2,960. Then Medicare pays nothing until expenses reach $4,700, the so-called doughnut hole, after which Medicare again pays about 95 percent.

Table 4.2	*Medicare Providers by Payments (in billions of dollars) and Persons Served (in millions), 2013*	
	Payments	**Persons Served**
Type of Provider		
Part A	$179.4	7.5
Inpatient hospital	129.5	6.5
Skilled nursing facility	28.2	1.8
Home health agency	6.8	1.7
Hospice	14.9	1.3
Part B	$166.6	33.2
Physician/DME	98.1	32.6
Outpatient	57.2	24.9
Home health agency	11.3	1.9

Source: *CMS Fast Facts* March 2015.

Changes under the Affordable Care Act phase in coverage of the "doughnut hole." By 2020, patients will pay only 25 percent of their prescription costs during that period. Because plan premiums, deductibles, copays, and formularies vary widely and change, enrollees are encouraged to review their plans and prescriptions during the fall open enrollment period to see if their current plan remains optimal for their needs. Through their websites and other information sources, the government attempts to assist individuals in making the best choice for their needs.

Reimbursement for Health Care Services

The federal government contracts with private insurance carriers to process payments and to act as intermediaries or carriers on behalf of the government. However, it is still the federal government that determines the level of reimbursement. Medicare was one of the earliest to begin adopting managed care strategies to control its costs.

Medicare uses a **prospective payment system (PPS)** to reimburse providers. The amount of the payment is determined prospectively, that is, before the patient receives services, and it is based on the patient's classification into a diagnostic-related group (DRG). Hospitals, skilled nursing facilities, and home health agencies are reimbursed on an "episode of care basis" using a PPS formula. Physicians are reimbursed on a fee-for-service basis. The fee schedule is based on the Resource-Based Relative Value schedule, which essentially pays more for specialty services. Medicare also sets limits on the total amount of payment.

The Affordable Care Act has numerous provisions regarding payments to physicians, hospitals, and other providers. The changes are intended to act as monetary incentives for productivity improvements and better primary care. Table 4.2 provides data that illustrate which health care providers are receiving reimbursement from Medicare and how many people were served. Under Part A, hospitals receive the majority of payments. Skilled nursing homes and hospices are receiving more payments now than 20 years ago. These additional payments reflect the needs of an elderly population whose life expectancy has improved. Part D benefits have expanded from $216 million in 2004 to $69.7 billion in 2013, again reflecting the needs of elderly people who are served by Medicare.

prospective payment system (PPS)
A payment system in which the amount of reimbursement is determined prior to the patient receiving services and is based on the patient's classification into a diagnostic-related group (DRG).

Medicaid

In 2013, Medicaid made up 15.4 percent of total national health expenditures; in 1966, the percentage was only 2.9 percent (CMS 2015). As you read at the beginning of the chapter, Medicaid has changed considerably under the Affordable Care Act and is now the largest source of public health coverage, covering nearly 70 million people (Paradise 2015). **Medicaid** is a transfer

Medicaid A federal and state program that funds health care primarily on the basis of the recipient's income.

program. It is funded by taxpayers' income tax payments to the government's general revenue. Congress then allocates these revenues to various national needs, such as health care. Like Medicare, Medicaid is also administered by the CMS. However, Medicaid is administered at the state level as well as at the federal level. This means that eligibility and coverage can and do differ from state to state.

To receive federal funds, states must provide Medicaid coverage to certain individuals. The state's Medicaid spending is matched by the federal government using a formula called the federal medical assistance percentage rate (FMAP). This rate is based on a state's per capita income as compared to the national average; in 2015, the rate varied from 50 percent to 73.6 percent.

Eligibility

The two major eligibility groups for Medicaid are poverty related and medically needy. Poverty-related Medicaid eligibility is determined by income and resources; it is designed to provide health care for those who otherwise would be unable to afford services. When an individual applies for Medicaid, the state evaluates that person's needs based on his or her income. Usually, if a person is eligible for supplemental security income (SSI) or temporary assistance for needy families (TANF), he or she is also eligible for Medicaid.

Medicaid is also available if the state determines that the individual is "medically needy." People who would otherwise not meet the income limit can use unpaid medical bills to lower, or spend down, their income. This eligibility category allows groups with large medical bills such as the elderly, pregnant women, children, and persons with disabilities to receive Medicaid benefits. The chapter profile provides more information about expanded eligibility.

Covered Benefits

Federal law specifies three categories of benefits. The first is benefits that all states' Medicaid programs must cover. This includes hospital and physician services. The second category of benefits is those the state may cover. This can include pharmaceutical, dental, and eye care coverage. The third group is benefits the state may not provide. For example, federal law prohibits using Medicaid funds to pay for abortions.

Table 4.3 provides information about the utilization of Medicaid services. It reveals some interesting discrepancies. Although children are the largest group of Medicaid recipients, they do not receive the majority of Medicaid spending. The majority of spending is for the elderly and people with disabilities, even though they are only a quarter of the recipients.

States have used this type of data to determine what benefits they can provide. A trade-off between the cost of some services and the number of

Table 4.3	*Medicaid Recipients and Payments, 2011*	
	Recipients	**Payments**
Total	68 million	$397.6 billion
Elderly	9%	21%
Disabled	15%	42%
Adults	27%	15%
Children	48%	21%

Source: Paradise, J. *Medicaid moving forward*. March 2015. The Kaiser Commission on Medicaid and the Uninsured, Figure 2.

people receiving benefits creates difficult decisions for state governments. The latest health reform law mandates states to reduce the numbers of their uninsured.

Reimbursement for Health Care Services

Medicaid reimburses providers on a fee-for-service/episode-of-care basis. Medicaid has managed care options in the same way Medicare has, and the majority of the Medicaid population is in managed care.

States are required to use a public process to determine their Medicaid reimbursement rates. However, many providers feel the rates are too low to make their participation in the program financially worthwhile. Under the Affordable Care Act, reimbursements to physicians who provide primary care services were increased to 100 percent of the Medicare rate for a period of time. Physicians and nursing homes are not required to accept Medicaid patients, which may limit a patient's ability to choose what provider he or she would prefer.

CHIP

An additional federal health insurance program was created in 1997 as part of the Balanced Budget Act. The **Children's Health Insurance Program (CHIP)** covers targeted low-income children whose parents do not qualify for Medicaid yet are unable to afford private health insurance. Children under the age of 19, including the unborn, are eligible. Each state operates its own plan, with a combination of federal and state funding. States had three options to achieve the objective of the program: they could choose to expand Medicaid coverage, they could set up a separate child health program, or they could combine the two options (Centers for Medicare & Medicaid Services 2004). States have continued to expand eligibility under the Affordable Care Act and changes to Medicaid eligibility, so that a child might be eligible for coverage under both programs depending on state of residency. In 2014, there were 8 million children enrolled in CHIP, 36.1 million in Medicaid, and

Children's Health Insurance Program (CHIP) A federal program that targets low-income children whose parents do not qualify for Medicaid, yet are unable to afford private health insurance.

43.6 million in both. Total expenditures for the CHIP program were $13.5 billion in 2013 (CMS 2015).

Waste, Fraud, and Abuse

Waste, fraud, and abuse of the Medicare and Medicaid programs are a serious concern and cost millions of dollars every year. The Affordable Care Act provided additional financial resources to fight fraud, increased federal sentencing guidelines, and required provider screening and enhanced oversight of new providers. A database to share information across states' and federal programs has been developed (www.stopmedicarefraud.gov). The Affordable Care Act is not the first time the government has addressed this problem. Provisions in the Health Insurance Portability and Accountability Act (HIPAA) legislation give the government greater authority to investigate and punish fraud. The Department of Health and Human Services and the Department of Justice developed joint fraud strike forces that have obtained indictments of more than 500 individuals and organizations for more than a billion dollars of billing fraud. Civil penalties include substantial fines; criminal penalties include imprisonment. Realistically, the most significant penalty is exclusion from the Medicare or Medicaid program.

Fraud occurs in a number of ways. Fraud may be committed intentionally to obtain payments the provider is not otherwise entitled to receive. For example, a provider might submit a claim for a service that was never provided or might submit the claim under a different code to receive a higher rate of reimbursement (called *upcoding*). Fraud is sometimes the result of good intentions. For example, when a sympathetic practitioner knows a service the patient needs is not covered, the practitioner may be tempted to code the service so it will be covered. Even with good intentions, this is still fraud. The Office of the Inspector General identifies fraud in Medicare Part D prescription drugs, Medicare home health benefits, Medicaid personal care services, durable medical equipment, behavioral health, and ambulance services as areas for potential fraud (Office of the Inspector General [OIG] 2015).

self-referral arrangements Health care providers are prohibited under federal law from referring patients to laboratories or other health services in which they have a financial interest.

Other federal legislation prohibits kickbacks and **self-referral arrangements**. The legislation prevents health care providers from making health care decisions based on the financial benefits they could receive, which include payments to induce referrals. Under Stark I, if a physician or his or her immediate family owns a clinical laboratory, the physician may not make referrals to that lab facility. Stark II is even broader and prohibits the physician from referrals to "designated health services" where there is a financial interest. "Designated health services" include clinical laboratories, physical and occupational therapy, radiology, equipment and supplies, and home health services. If the physician has made a prohibited referral, the health services may not bill Medicare for payment.

Most health care organizations have chosen to meet this challenge by implementing **compliance programs**. A strong compliance program ensures that all claims submitted for payment have appropriate documentation. In addition, it is particularly important that providers receive regular training to stay current with Medicare and Medicaid regulations. Compliance programs are mandatory under the Patient Protection and Affordable Care Act.

compliance programs A program that is implemented in a business to ensure the business stays in compliance with current legislation, especially changes in the Medicare and Medicaid programs.

Programs for Special Populations

In addition to the programs already described in this chapter, the federal government provides health insurance programs for two additional groups. One is government workers, and the other is military personnel.

Federal employees' health care needs are covered by the **Federal Employees Health Benefits Program (FEHBP)**. The Office of Personnel Management (OPM) administers the program, which is the human resources department of the federal government. The FEHBP is an employer-sponsored health insurance program. This makes it more similar to the insurance options described in Chapter 3 than to the government programs such as Medicare and Medicaid described in this chapter.

Federal Employees Health Benefits Program (FEHBP) An employer-sponsored health insurance program available to employees of the federal government.

Federal employees, families, retirees, and survivors are covered under the FEHBP program, making it one of the largest employer-sponsored health insurance programs in the world. Enrollees can choose from a wide selection of plans, including fee-for-service, point-of-service, or HMOs. Because the federal government is a purchaser of insurance, it has the ability to influence what types of programs are offered and what level of premium is charged. The federal government began exploring managed care options in the 1970s, leading many other employer-sponsored health insurance programs to follow suit.

Health care coverage for military personnel is another government payment program. **TRICARE** is the Department of Defense's health insurance program for eligible beneficiaries in the uniformed services. The TRICARE program (formerly known as CHAMPUS) has a variety of managed care options such as HMOs, preferred providers, and fee-for-service. Care is provided by civilian health care providers who contract with TRICARE to become a preferred provider. Under certain circumstances, a military treatment facility may be the provider for TRICARE-covered services.

TRICARE A health insurance program offered by the Department of Defense to military personnel.

Retired military personnel may also be eligible for Medicare; there are regulations that cover which insurance program will pay for what services. However, neither Medicare nor TRICARE covers long-term care needs such as a nursing home.

As you'll read elsewhere, the federal government also takes the role of a health care provider through the Veterans Administration hospitals. The federal government's role in the TRICARE program is as a purchaser of insurance.

Workers' Compensation Insurance

workers' compensation A program that provides health care benefits to employees who are injured on the job.

Employees are another category of people who can receive health care benefits under a government-administered program called **workers' compensation**. Workers' compensation acts were designed to eliminate the need for an employee to sue the employer for negligence when the employee was injured in the workplace. In return for giving up the right to sue for damages, employees gain the certainty of compensation at a predetermined level.

The process is straightforward. When an employee is injured, he or she files a claim with the state government agency. In most states, this agency is called the workers' compensation commission or the workers' compensation board. The employee must prove that the injury was work related. The government agency determines if the claim is legitimate and what benefits the employee is entitled to receive. Benefits are predetermined based on the type of injury and the amount of time the employee will be unable to work. If the employee is denied benefits for some reason, he or she can appeal the decision. However, the employee cannot sue the employer unless the employer intentionally caused the injury.

Workers' compensation is funded by employers. Depending on state law, the employer either pays for workers' compensation insurance or self-insures by making payments into a contingency fund. An incentive to maintain a safe workplace is built into the system: employers' premium rates drop if they have low numbers of accidents. New Jersey, South Carolina, and Texas have designed voluntary plans that allow the employer to decide if it will participate in the system or be open to negligence claims by the injured employee.

Like all insurance plans, workers' compensation is vulnerable to fraud and abuse. There are cases of employees claiming injuries that don't exist or were not work related. Back injuries, in particular, are prone to false claims. There are also cases of employees deliberately injuring themselves on the job in order to recover.

Issues for Government Payment Programs

The role of federal and state governments in providing health care services is controversial. Who should be eligible, what services should be provided, and how providers should be compensated are ongoing issues that governments must address. In these times of rising costs, the government must be both a good steward of taxpayers' money and at the same time provide health care as broadly as possible.

Eligibility and Benefits

As you've seen in this chapter, the eligibility and benefits issues go hand in hand. Especially at the state level, Medicaid programs have used different models to decide what services to provide. Decisions to expand access (prescription drugs) or limit access (abortions) are often based on political, rather than medical, factors. Government programs continue to provide care for the elderly and the poor. The Affordable Care Act has expanded care, especially to those who were uninsured.

Payments

As one of the largest purchasers of health care services, the government has implemented strategies to manage costs. Through size alone, it can force providers to accept the payment program it offers. However, as seen with the Medicaid program, where providers feel that the financial incentives are inadequate, they will opt out of the program. Cost savings therefore translate into reduced access for certain categories of patients. The Affordable Care Act requires a number of demonstration projects aimed at special populations and creates oversight boards to monitor costs.

Career Profile: Government Agencies

This chapter has focused on describing various government programs that provide health care services and payments, how much the services cost, and who is covered. But don't forget that every one of these programs is a potential place of employment. In fact, federal and state governments are the largest employers in the overall economy.

The www.usajobs.gov website is a central clearinghouse for federal jobs and is searchable in many ways. Of particular interest to students is the capacity to search by jobs related to college major and by jobs for recent graduates (the Pathways Project). You can also search by agency or location.

The Centers for Medicare & Medicaid Services, for example, hire positions as varied as secretaries, accountants, actuaries, nurses, programmers, social scientists, and managers. A secretary in the office of a Center Director provides administrative support and office management for the director, deputy director, and group directors. This type of position requires experience, and the pay ranges from $47,684 to $68,465. A Health Insurance Specialist might provide technical assistance and reports to management on Medicare Advantage and Medicare Health Plans to ensure those programs deliver adequate levels of service to program enrollees; a master's degree and Medicare experience is required, and the salary ranges from $57,000 to $90,000. From this position you can move up into a supervisory position. The Director of the Investigations and Audits Group is an executive-level position that manages investigative and enforcement activities. The director oversees field offices of the Center for Program Integrity and works with law enforcement agencies to develop cases. A high level of experience is required for an executive position, which is reflected in a pay level of $121,000 to $183,000.

Summary

Many people's health care costs are paid by government programs. Medicare provides benefits primarily to the elderly. Approximately 55 million people receive Medicare; the program costs the government $585 billion. Medicare pays for hospitalization, regular medical care, and, if elected, prescription drug coverage. Medicaid is a program primarily for the poor. Of the 68 million receiving Medicaid, almost half are children. However, the bulk of Medicaid spending is for the elderly, particularly for long-term care. Additional government programs address the needs of children and government/military employees. Workers' compensation is funded by employers, is administered by the government, and covers work-related injuries.

Questions for Review

1. List three ways a person becomes eligible for Medicare benefits.
2. What is the difference in coverage between Part A and Part B of Medicare? What is covered under Part D?
3. How is a person eligible for Medicaid?
4. What is CHIP?
5. Who pays for workers' compensation?

Questions for Discussion

1. What groups do you believe are not being served under the current system of government health care programs? How should they be served? What services should be provided? How will government pay for the services?
2. Should Medicare fund long-term care, regardless of income?
3. As discussed earlier in the chapter, the "doughnut hole" was designed to keep the cost of Medicare Part D manageable. Has this objective been achieved? Are there better ways to manage costs?
4. Should the government require providers to accept Medicaid patients?
5. Review the provisions for Medicaid eligibility in your own state. Has the Affordable Care Act made a difference to the number of uninsured?
6. Do the mechanisms for preventing fraud and abuse seem adequate? How could they be improved?
7. Can an employer prevent fraudulent claims by employees of work-related injuries?

Chapter References

Centers for Medicare & Medicaid Services. March 2015. *CMS Fast Facts.* _____. 2004. *Program information on Medicaid and State Children's Health Insurance Program (SCHIP).* Baltimore: Author.

Office of the Inspector General (OIG). June 18, 2015. *National health care fraud take-down.* Washington, DC: U.S. Department of Health and Human Services.

Paradise, J. March 2015. *Medicaid moving forward.* Washington, DC: The Kaiser Commission on Medicaid and the Uninsured.

Stop Medicare Fraud (www.stopmedicarefraud.gov).

TRICARE (http://tricare.mil).

U.S. Census Bureau. *Statistical abstract of the United States: 2010.*

For Additional Information

Centers for Medicare & Medicaid Services (www.cms.gov).

Healthcare.gov

Medicare, The Official U.S. Government Site for Medicare (www.medicare.gov).

5

Health Care Providers

Physicians and Nurses

Learning Objectives

After reading this chapter, you should be able to:

1. Describe the roles of the physician and nurse in providing health care services.

2. Compare and contrast the different types of physicians and nurses.

3. Describe the demographic characteristics of physicians and nurses.

4. Outline the education and training process of physicians and nurses.

5. Identify the requirements for licensure, and explain the difference between licensure and certification.

6. Identify employment settings for physicians and nurses.

7. Describe the major issues facing the professions of physician and nurse.

A Family Practitioner

Carrie Hunter, MD, advises that the best way for people to understand what the life of a family practitioner is really like is to tag along for a week. They would see her interacting with patients and checking on her patients at the hospital, but they'd also see her on the phone, ordering tests and supplies and generally checking on things, or hitting the books and the Internet to investigate a patient's problem. "Even when you're not at work, you really still are. Sometimes you're the only one who can do what needs to be done for your patient."

Hunter is one of 18 family practitioners and 4 internists in group practice in Jonesboro, Arkansas. Her days start around 7:30 or 8 A.M. at the hospital. She usually has only two or three patients in the hospital, which is the way she likes it. "I want to treat them in the clinic so they don't have to be admitted." But if one of her patients has been admitted with pneumonia, for example, she'll order fluids and antibiotics. When she goes to the hospital, she checks on the blood work and X-rays she ordered. "Then I rely on the nurses to check on my patients." Sometimes she'll swing by again at lunch or in the evening.

By 9 A.M. she's at the clinic. She schedules patients every 15 minutes, preferring to have her mornings full and work through lunch rather than to stay late in the evenings. New patients or longer procedures such as Pap smears and lesion removals are scheduled for 30 minutes. Three times a week, she spends half of her day in the practice's urgent care clinic. The clinic is open weekends and takes patients without appointments. They aren't necessarily even her patients. The clinic sees about 60 patients a day and up to 100 during flu season. "We get overflow from the local pediatricians for colds and strep throat, and even people who should have probably gone directly to the ER."

"The best part about my job is really getting to see yourself making a difference," says Hunter. "In family practice you do routine illness, and you follow patients

Introduction

In the United States today, almost 16 million people are employed in the health care industry. Physicians and nurses make up about a quarter of all health care employees. Patient care is delivered by a team of professionals that includes physicians, nurses, and other clinical providers. The patient care team is supported by non-clinical staff and business professionals. Physicians play an important role in the delivery of health care services. According to the National Center for Health Statistics, there were over a billion visits to physicians' offices in 2010. Of all the health professions, nursing employs the largest number of people, with more than 3 million jobs in 2012 (Bureau of Labor Statistics, RNs 2014–15). In this chapter, you will learn about the roles of the physicians and nurses as part of a health care provider team, where they work, how they are trained and licensed, and the issues facing these providers as the health care environment continues to change. The following chapter addresses the other clinical and non-clinical providers.

with blood pressure, diabetes, and heart disease. You see them for a long time and get to know their whole family." One patient even brought a birthday gift for her daughter.

"Primary care is one-third psychiatry. It's counseling as well as technical knowledge." One of the frustrations is dealing with patients who aren't taking care of themselves. "Smoking and alcohol are big problems. Some patients just want you to fix them with a pill so they can keep doing what they're doing." Hunter notes that sometimes it's hard to be nice and supportive all day, every day when you see people who aren't at their best. Doctors internalize, she says: "Where do you go with all that bad stuff?"

Hunter recently took the exam to be board certified in family medicine. She considers it good review because she has to recertify every 7 years. Each year they get review modules, so she's up-to-date on the latest treatments for blood pressure or cholesterol. "Every day I see at least one thing I don't know about. I do research that day—either in my books or on the Internet. And I talk to my partners."

One of the challenges Hunter anticipates is the desire of female physicians to have a lifestyle where they can take care of both their patients and their families. All her female preceptors in medical school were career oriented and had never married or were divorced and childless. "All that has changed," Hunter notes. "Female physicians are like me. We're having children, and we want both—a life and a practice. If we can do both, then the men can back off too."

Hunter says, "I'm glad I do what I do. It's interesting work and I make a good living. The downside is there's no control over the hours." What she hopes to do in the next phase of her career is focus mostly on the clinic and women's health issues. "I'd like more of my patients to be the 18- to 45-year-old women. Sometimes they have trouble relating with a male physician. It's something I'd be good at."

The Physician's Role in Health Care Delivery

The role of physicians is to diagnose and treat the illnesses of their patients. When a physician sees a patient who has an injury or is ill, the physician must first identify the problem or diagnose the illness. The process begins with the physician obtaining the patient's **medical history** and performing a physical examination. To aid in the diagnosis, the physician may perform or order diagnostic tests and then interpret the results. Once the physician has made a diagnosis, treatment for the patient will be prescribed or administered. In addition, physicians give their patients advice about preventive health care and make suggestions about diet and hygiene that will help the patients live healthier lives (Bureau of Labor Statistics, Physicians 2014–15).

medical history The record of a patient's health, physicians' visits, symptoms, prescribed treatments, regular medications, and family medical history.

Types of Physicians and Medical Specialties

Physicians are either doctors of medicine (as indicated by the abbreviation MD after their name) or doctors of osteopathy (as indicated by the abbreviation DO). MDs practice **allopathic medicine**, which means they fight disease by using standard treatments, including surgery and drugs. Although the DO may use these same treatments, DOs practice **osteopathic medicine**, where a special emphasis is placed on understanding the body's musculoskeletal system and on providing preventive and holistic care that considers the relationship between the body, the mind, and the emotions of the patient (Bureau of Labor Statistics, Physicians 2014–15).

During medical school, students are exposed to the many medical specialties. In part, this exposure is designed to help them decide what area of medicine they would like to focus on. Physicians are usually described either as primary care providers or as specialists.

allopathic medicine A process of treating disease by using standard treatments, such as surgery and drugs.

osteopathic medicine A process of treating patients by providing preventive and holistic care.

Primary Care

More than half of DOs and a third of MDs are **primary care physicians**. A primary care physician sees the same patients regularly for preventive care and to treat a variety of common health problems. The main areas of primary care are internal medicine, general and family practice, and pediatrics (Bureau of Labor Statistics, Physicians 2014–15).

Internal medicine focuses on problems associated with the body's organs. An internist is trained to diagnose and treat common problems and diseases of the heart, blood, eyes, ears, skin, kidneys, and the digestive, respiratory, and vascular systems. The patients an internist treats are usually adults, although internists often treat children with diabetes or chronic gastrointestinal diseases.

General and family practitioners diagnose and treat a wide variety of illnesses in patients of all ages. This requires a range of training that includes internal medicine, obstetrics and gynecology, and pediatrics. Special emphasis is placed on comprehensive health care of the family as a group.

Pediatricians focus their efforts on a particular group of patients: children. It is the norm for pediatricians to provide preventive health care for children through regular checkups and immunizations. However, they also diagnose and treat infections, injuries, and serious illnesses as needed by their patients.

primary care physicians The physician who sees a patient regularly for routine and preventive care.

internal medicine An area of medicine that focuses on the body's organs, such as the heart, eyes, ears, kidneys, and the digestive, respiratory, and vascular systems.

general and family practitioner Physician who focuses on providing comprehensive health care to patients of all ages.

pediatrician A physician who focuses on providing care to children.

Specialty Care

Health insurance coverage usually requires that the patient first see the primary care physician for diagnosis and treatment. If required, the primary care physician then refers the patient to a specialist, a physician who is an expert in that particular medical field. Table 5.1 lists some of the typical specialties and their definitions.

Table 5.1	*Medical Specialties*
Allergy and immunology	Abnormal responses or acquired hypersensitivity to substances
Anesthesiology	Administration of medications to cause loss of feeling
Cardiovascular diseases	Diseases of the heart and blood vessels
Dermatology	Diseases of the skin
Emergency medicine	Acute illness or injury
Gastroenterology	Diseases and disorders of the stomach and intestine
Neurology	Diseases of the brain and nervous system
Obstetrics and gynecology	Pregnancy, childbirth, and diseases of the female reproductive organs
Pathology	Diagnosis of disease by studying changes in organs, tissues, and cells
Psychiatry	Diseases and disorders of the mind
Pulmonary diseases	Diseases of the lungs
Radiology	Use of X-rays and radiation to diagnose and treat illness
Urology	Diseases of the kidney, bladder, or urinary system

If the patient needs an operation to treat the injury or disease, the patient is referred to a **surgeon**. Most surgeons specialize in a particular type of surgery; these include orthopedics (skeletal system and associated organs), ophthalmology (eye), neurological (brain and nervous system), and plastic and reconstructive surgery (Bureau of Labor Statistics, Physicians 2014–15). During surgery, the patient will also need the services of an anesthesiologist.

surgeon A physician who performs operations.

Characteristics of U.S. Physicians

According to the Department of Labor, 691,400 physicians were in active practice in 2012 (Bureau of Labor Statistics, Physicians 2014–15). The demographic data indicate that the profession has slowly changed from one that only white men could enter to one with more opportunities for women and minorities. For example, in 1980 less than 12 percent of physicians were women; in 2014, more than 35 percent are women. Asians represent the largest group of minorities (about 12%), followed by Hispanics (about 5%) and African Americans (about 4%; AAMC 2014).

Because the population of the United States has become more diverse, it is important that the physician population also continue to diversify. Some studies show that patients report greater comfort and satisfaction with a physician whose ethnicity and gender mirror their own (Association of American Medical Colleges [AAMC] 2014). A diversified physician population may also improve patient access. Minority and female physicians are more likely to practice in primary care and to serve disadvantaged populations.

Employment and Earnings of Physicians

Our image of a physician working as a solo practitioner is more a product of art and television than reality. Only 21 percent are solo practice owners, and 17 percent have an ownership share in a practice. About 14 percent are employed by a privately owned practice; almost 21 percent were employed by hospitals (Bureau of Labor Statistics, Physicians 2014–15). The others worked in the government, with the Veterans Administration (VA) Hospital or the public health service of Health and Human Services (HHS), for example. The physicians who are not in active practice are teachers, administrators, and researchers. A small number are not involved in medicine at all.

hospitalists
Physicians who focus on providing care to hospitalized patients.

The employment of physicians called **hospitalists** is a growing trend. The traditional model was for a primary care physician to admit patients to the hospital where she or he had staff privileges; in this model, the physician is not an employee of the hospital. In the hospitalist model, the hospitalist provides care for the admitted patient; the hospitalist is employed by the hospital. Close to 44,000 physicians are employed as hospitalists; 72 percent of hospitals now employ hospitalists, up from 29 percent in 2003. The growth in the number of hospitalists is driven in part by physician practice factors such as declining revenues and desire for work–life balance and in part by hospital factors such as shortages of primary care physicians, emergency department coverage, and restrictions on residents' hours (Society for Hospital Medicine [SHM] 2014).

It is typical for most physicians to work long, irregular hours. In 2014, 49 percent of physicians reported they worked more than 50 hours per week; 13 percent work between 60 and 70 hours each week (AMA 2014). One advantage of working in a group practice is that the heavy workload is shared by more physicians.

Because the health care industry is expected to continue expanding, the Department of Labor forecasts that the need for physicians will grow by more than 18 percent through 2022 (Bureau of Labor Statistics, Physicians 2014–15). Some specialties are oversupplied; due to the aging of the American population, job prospects are better in specialties such as cardiology or radiology. Job prospects are also good for those willing to relocate to rural areas where there aren't as many physicians. Some states have tried to attract recent graduates to rural areas by offering to repay their student loans.

Although the workload is sometimes viewed as a disadvantage by those considering the profession, the salary is an advantage. Physicians have among the highest earnings of any profession. The median net income for physicians in primary care is $220,942 per year, according to the 2012 Medical Group Management Association's Physician Compensation and Production Survey. For many physicians, earnings are much higher. Income level varies by number of years in practice, geographic region, hours worked, and specialty. For example, median net income for specialty fields is $396,233.

Education and Training

The education and training required to become a physician has two components. The formal education component consists of an undergraduate degree from a university or college, followed by graduate medical education in medical school. The training component occurs on the job.

The first step toward becoming a physician is an undergraduate degree, usually with a pre-med or science major. The second part of a physician's formal education occurs in medical school. Medical school looks the way it does today thanks to the efforts of the AMA to move training from an apprenticeship style to a scientific university-based education. The Flexner Report in 1910 recommended what has become the current model of medical education: a 4-year program, with 2 years of basic science and 2 years of clinical experience (Beck 2004). Medical school curricula have continued to change as the medical field has changed. More students are exposed to complementary and alternative medicine. Students are also taught to care for culturally diverse populations. Today there are 171 medical schools in the United States—141 teach allopathic medicine and award the MD; 30 teach osteopathic medicine and award the DO (www. aamc.org). Admission to medical school is very competitive, with less than half of the applicants being accepted. Of these, about 47 percent are women, 7.1 percent African American, 19 percent Asian, and 5.8 percent Hispanic. Ninety-six percent graduate (AAMC 2014).

The final stage of a physician's preparation is **residency**, now referred to as Graduate Medical Education (previously called internship and residency). It is paid on-the-job training. Depending on the specialty, residency can last from 1 to 7 years (www.acgme.org).

residency The last stage of physician training. After medical school, the student completes on-the-job training in his or her specialty.

Medical school tuition and fees have continued to increase: the median cost of attendance for the class of 2015 is between $227,000 and $298,000. Because medical school is so expensive, 84 percent of students borrow money so that they can attend. According to the Association of American Medical Colleges (AAMC), the average debt for a 2014 graduate is $176,348; 79 percent of graduates carry more than $100,000 of debt, and 43 percent owe more than $200,000 (AAMC 2014).

The increased cost of medical school creates several concerns. The first is an increase in undesirable physician behaviors such as moonlighting and depression. A second concern is that the cost will disproportionately affect minority students, leading to a decrease in diversity. Finally, there is concern that students with high levels of debt may decide not to practice in the lower paying areas of primary care or to work in underserved areas.

Licensure and Certification

The final step is licensure. Every state sets its own requirements for licensure; however, the three standard requirements are graduating from medical school, completing 1 to 7 years of residency, and passing a licensing exam. The U.S.

Medical Practice Act State legislation that sets out the requirements for physician licensure in that state.

reciprocity agreement An agreement between two states in which each accepts the professional licensing requirements of the other.

CME (Continuing Medical Education) The state requirement that physicians receive a certain amount of additional training and education to remain licensed.

board certification A physician may become board certified by completing additional years of residency in the specialty and passing an exam.

Medical Licensing Examination (USMLE) is a three-step exam required for licensure in the United States (www.nbme.org). Only a handful of states require criminal background checks or fingerprinting of applicants. The state's specific requirements for licensure are set out in its **Medical Practice Act**, and the license is granted by the state's Board of Medical Examiners. Physicians may only practice medicine in a state where they have a license. To practice in another state, the physician must obtain a license in that state. The state may have a **reciprocity agreement**, which means it accepts the licensing requirements of the first state.

To stay licensed, the physician must pay an annual renewal fee. States also require that physicians stay current in the field by completing additional education, called **CME (Continuing Medical Education)**. Although state requirements may vary, the standard requirement is 75 hours of CME over a 3-year period. Physicians who do not meet these requirements can lose their licenses and hospital privileges.

The state's Medical Practice Act specifies the conditions when a state may suspend or revoke a physician's license. The conditions generally include unprofessional conduct, commission of a crime, or personal incapacity to perform one's duties. The licensing board provides notice to the physician and performs an investigation before a decision is made to revoke the license. The Board may choose to suspend the physician's license during this period if it believes that a dangerous situation exists.

Unlike licensure, **board certification** is voluntary and a way for the physician to indicate that he or she has additional training and skill in a particular area of medicine. To obtain board certification in any of 24 areas, physicians must complete the required years of residency in that specialty and then pass an exam. When these requirements are successfully completed, physicians may refer to themselves as "board certified." Others refer to the physician as a "diplomat" of that particular board. The two organizations that control board certification are the American Board of Medical Specialties and the American Osteopathic Association.

The Nurse's Role in Health Care Delivery

As you can see from Table 5.2, there are a number of definitions of nursing; however, all include some aspect of caring for the patient as a whole. A brief definition of the nurse's role is that nurses "take care of people."

"Taking care of people" can include interviewing, examining, and evaluating patients when they first seek health care services. It may progress to providing treatment and care as the patient receives health care services. It may also include working with other health care professionals and referring the patient elsewhere for other services. It includes patient advocacy. The actual day-to-day tasks performed by a nurse are usually determined by the work setting. In addition to the traditional role of direct patient care, nurses' roles have expanded to include disease prevention and health promotion.

Table 5.2	*Definitions of Nursing*

The "Practice of Nursing" means assisting individuals or groups to maintain or attain optimal health, implementing a strategy of care to accomplish defined goals, and evaluating responses to care and treatment.
Source: Model Practice Act, National Council of State Boards of Nursing, 1994.

The first level nurse is responsible for planning, providing, and evaluating nursing care in all settings for the promotion of health, prevention of illness, care of the sick, and rehabilitation; and functions as a member of the health team.
Source: International Council of Nurses, 1973.

Nursing is the diagnosis and treatment of human responses to actual or potential health problems.
Source: American Nurses Association Social Policy Statement, 1995.

The essential components of professional nursing are care, cure, and coordination.
Source: American Nurses Association, First Position Paper on Education, Committee on Nursing Education, 1965.

<To have> charge of the personal health of somebody . . . and what nursing has to do . . . is to put the patient in the best condition for nature to act upon him.
Source: Florence Nightingale, Notes on Nursing: What It Is and What It Is Not (London: Harrison and Sons, 1859).

The **nursing process** is an organizing framework that provides a systematic method to deliver patient care (Harrington and Terry 2012). The five stages in the nursing process are assessment, diagnosis, care planning, implementation, and outcome evaluation. The process begins with assessment, or the gathering of information. Information can come directly from the patient or from friends, family, and other health care providers. The next step is a nursing diagnosis. The information that has been gathered is reviewed, the problem identified, and a nursing diagnosis made. The North American Nursing Diagnosis Association (NANDA) has developed a classification and formatting system for nursing diagnoses.

Based on the nursing diagnosis, care is planned. Planning actually involves two steps: writing client goals and planning interventions to achieve the goals. There are 490 identified outcomes that are responsive to nursing care; these are classified on the **Nursing Outcomes Classification (NOC)** (Moorhead, Johnson, Mass, and Swanson 2012). In the **Nursing Interventions Classification (NIC)**, 554 interventions are identified. These are the nursing treatments of choice for each nursing diagnosis (Bulechek, Butcher, Dochteman, and Wagner 2012). Then the plan is implemented. Finally, the outcome is evaluated. In actuality, evaluation is ongoing so that modifications can be made to the care plan.

nursing process An organizing framework that provides a systematic method to deliver patient care.

Nursing Outcomes Classification (NOC) A list of 490 identified outcomes that are responsive to nursing care.

Nursing Interventions Classification (NIC) A list of 554 interventions that are the nursing treatments of choice for each nursing diagnosis.

Characteristics of U.S. Nurses

Most of our images of the nursing profession come from the media, yet not all of these impressions are accurate. The media usually portrays nurses as young females. Of the more than 3 million people employed in nursing, it's estimated that 90 percent are women; however, men are increasingly choosing nursing as a profession. Less than 5 percent of nurses are under the age of 25; the average age of RNs is 45 (Health Resources and Services Administration [HRSA] 2013).

Nursing continues to be a predominantly white profession. More than 75 percent of RNs are white, but like other health occupations, the number of minority nurses has increased. African Americans represent about 10 percent of RNs, Asians about 8 percent, and Hispanics about 5 percent.

Types of Nurses

To the general public, a nurse is a nurse is a nurse. Contrary to this misperception, there are significant differences in the types of nurses. The differences include the tasks/responsibilities, the extent of training and education, and the requirements for professional licensing.

Nurses' Assistants and Aides

nurse's aide Health care worker who provides the most basic level of patient care, such as feeding and hygiene.

The nursing assistant or aide is not actually a nurse at all. In some health care settings, **nurses' aides** and home health aides are referred to as NAs and CNAs, depending on whether certification has been obtained. In 2012, there were about 1.5 million nurses' aides (Bureau of Labor Statistics, Nursing Assistants 2014–15).

Under the supervision of an RN, NAs provide the most basic level of patient care. Basic care includes physical care of the patient, such as feeding and hygiene. An NA answers call bells, serves meals, and makes beds. The NA may help the patient get out of bed and walk and may escort the patient within the hospital or nursing facility. NAs also set up equipment and move supplies. In nursing homes, the NA is often the principal caregiver. In the home health setting, if they have taken advanced training, NAs may give oral medications to their patients (Sorrentino and Remmert 2013).

CNA (Certified Nursing Assistant) A nurse's aide who has received the credential of CNA.

NAs are trained on the job or complete a short course of study offered by the hospital or nursing home or by a community/technical college. An NA may obtain the credential of **CNA (Certified Nursing Assistant)**; not all states require certification. NAs are not required to obtain a state license, but some states do require registration. Federal guidelines require that home health aides whose employers receive Medicare reimbursement pass a competency test (Bureau of Labor Statistics, Nursing Assistants 2014–15).

licensed practical nurse (LPN) A nurse who has completed a state-approved program and passed a national exam. Generally, LPNs are supervised by RNs when providing patient care.

Licensed Practical or Licensed Vocational Nurse

The next level of care is provided by the **licensed practical nurse (LPN)** or the licensed vocational nurse (LVN). More than 738,000 LPNs were employed in 2012 (Bureau of Labor Statistics, LPNs 2014–15). The duties of the practical nurse include the basic bedside physical care of the patient. In addition to feeding patients and assisting with their personal hygiene, LPNs take vital signs, give medications and injections, and administer some IV medications.

Educational programs for LPNs last about a year. Ninety percent of programs are at technical/vocational schools or community colleges. The training includes both classroom and clinical experience. After completing their formal education program, LPNs must pass a national licensure exam to practice.

Registered Nurse

The majority (2.7 million in 2012) of nurses are **registered nurses (RNs)**. A higher level of care is provided by the RN. When performing direct patient care tasks, RNs observe, assess, and record symptoms, reactions, and progress. They may administer IV medication and blood. RNs perform patient assessments and plan care. As part of the nursing care plan developed and managed by the RN, the RN must instruct both the patient and the patient's family in proper care (Bureau of Labor Statistics, RNs 2014–15).

Some of the major differences between the LPN and the RN involve supervision, legal responsibilities, and IV therapy. The LPN and RN roles also vary in terms of the skill level required in communication, assessment, and client teaching (Harrington and Terry 2012). LPN training programs focus on the "how-to" of patient care, whereas RN education emphasizes understanding "why" (Hill and Howlett 2012).

The educational program for RNs is more complex than that for LPNs. RNs complete additional coursework toward an associate's degree, which includes additional clinical hours. Many community college offer bridge programs, designed for LPNs who wish to move up. RNs are encouraged to complete the **BSN (Bachelor of Science in Nursing)**. Like LPNs, to practice, RNs must pass a national licensure exam.

Additional promotions come from moving up a career ladder at a place of employment and assuming managerial responsibilities. RNs with the bachelor's or master's degree may choose a teaching career.

Advanced Practice Nurses

Advanced practice nurses provide their patients an even higher level of care. To become an advanced practice nurse, an RN must have a master's degree in a clinical specialty. A person can choose to become a **nurse practitioner (NP)**, a **clinical nurse specialist (CNS)**, a **certified nurse-midwife (CNM)**, or a **certified registered nurse anesthetist (CRNA)** (Blais and Hayes 2015).

There are currently more than 205,000 nurse practitioners in the United States (AANP 2015). NPs serve an important function in areas not adequately served by physicians such as rural communities and inner cities. They also are key health care providers for populations such as children in schools and the elderly. In these settings, NPs provide basic primary health care, including diagnosis and treatment of common acute illnesses. They can order and interpret X-rays and other laboratory tests. NPs can prescribe medications in all 50 states (including controlled substances in 49).

registered nurse (RN) A nurse who develops and manages a nursing care plan for a patient.

BSN (Bachelor of Science in Nursing) A bachelor's program that usually takes 4 years to complete.

advanced practice nurse A nurse who has obtained a master's degree in a clinical specialty.

nurse practitioner (NP) Advanced practice nurse who provides basic primary health care.

clinical nurse specialist (CNS) An advanced practice nurse who specializes in a field such as oncology, neonatal care, or mental health.

certified nurse-midwife (CNM) An advanced practice nurse who provides prenatal and postpartum care and delivers infants.

certified registered nurse anesthetist (CRNA) An advanced practice nurse who specializes in anesthesia.

The AANP reports that 97 percent of NPs prescribe medications, averaging 19 prescriptions per day. Certification is available for NPs who wish to specialize in acute, adult, family, gerontological, or pediatric care (Blais and Hayes 2015).

Instead of focusing on primary care, nurse practitioners may choose the role of clinical nurse specialist (CNS). Some of the specialties for practice include cardiac, oncology, neonatal, obstetrics/gynecology, pediatrics, neurological nursing, and psychiatric/mental health care.

Certified nurse-midwives (CNMs) and certified registered nurse anesthetists (CRNAs) are two additional areas of specialization. More than 11,018 CNMs in clinical practice provide prenatal care to healthy women, deliver babies, and provide postpartum care for their patients. Reproductive care and primary care are main responsibilities. Many of the patients served by CNMs are considered "vulnerable" because of their age, socioeconomic status, ethnicity, education, or location of residency (www.acnm.org). Since 2010, a graduate degree is required to enter midwifery practice.

The more than 48,000 CRNAs in the United States play a central role in anesthesiology. According to the American Association of Nurse Anesthetists, nurse anesthetists administered approximately 34 million anesthetics in 2013. In nearly 100 percent of rural U.S. hospitals, the CRNA is the sole provider of anesthetics (www.aana.com). Unlike other areas of nursing, this is not a female-dominated specialty; more than 40 percent of nurse anesthetists are men.

Education and Training

At all levels, nursing education has two components: classroom instruction and **supervised clinical experience**. As nursing has evolved as a profession, the level of education and training has shifted from primarily on-the-job training to formal college-based education. Although there are a few **diploma programs** still offered by hospitals, the majority of RN programs are offered at the **ADN (associate degree in nursing)** level and the BSN level (Bureau of Labor Statistics, RN 2014–15). Either degree qualifies a licensed nurse for an entry-level staff position. However, advancement opportunities into management positions may require the bachelor's degree.

The profession is encouraging nurses to complete bachelor's, master's, and even doctoral degrees in nursing. Currently about 55 percent of nurses have bachelor's degrees or higher. Enrollment and graduation rates from BSN programs have continued to rise, but growth is constrained by lack of faculty and clinical sites. Enrollment in graduate programs increased 67 percent between 2007 and 2011. Higher level degrees are required for teaching and research positions. Graduate training is required for management-level nursing positions and for advanced practitioner patient care.

Licensure

In each state, the **State Board of Nursing** (or its equivalent) specifies what educational, clinical, and licensure requirements are necessary to practice in that state. **Nurse Practice Acts** contain the states' requirements for practice. Although

---

supervised clinical experience Nursing students obtain hands-on experience with patients as part of their education.

diploma program Hospitals used to provide on-the-job training programs for nurses and award a diploma on completion. Very few diploma programs still exist.

ADN (associate degree in nursing) An associate's program typically takes 2 years to complete and is usually offered by a community college.

State Board of Nursing Each state has an agency that oversees the profession and accredits educational programs.

Nurse Practice Act State legislation that sets out the requirements for nurse licensure in the state.

they vary from state to state in their details, practice acts generally define the scope of nursing practice, control who may use nursing titles, specify educational requirements, and identify causes for disciplinary action (Harrington and Terry 2012).

All 50 states require that nurses be and remain licensed in order to practice. Once a nurse has finished the educational program requirements, the next step is to take the national registry exam (NCLEX). At each level of practice, there is a separate licensure exam. If the exam is passed, then licensure by the state to practice follows, and the title LPN or RN can be used.

The continuing education requirements for nurses vary. Generally, the more specialized the practice, the more likely it is that continuing education is required to maintain licensure or certification. Like physicians, nurses are subject to disciplinary actions. They have to stay in good standing or risk having their license not renewed or even revoked.

Employment Options for Nurses

Everywhere health care services are provided, you'll find nurses. The work nurses do in hospitals, offices, long-term care, home health, public health, and other settings is described in the following sections. The salaries earned by LPNs and RNs and the percentage of each type of nurse working in different health care setting are presented in Table 5.3.

Hospitals

The entry-level position for an RN is **staff nurse**. Staff nurses provide bedside care and carry out medical regimens. They also supervise LPNs and NAs. A staff nurse is usually assigned to one area such as surgery, maternity, pediatrics, emergency department, or intensive care.

staff nurse An entry-level position for a nurse.

With more experience, an RN can be promoted to a **nurse supervisor** position. Nurse supervisors plan work schedules and assign duties for their area. They also provide training for other nurses. They visit patients to observe the patients' care. Maintaining records and ordering supplies are among the nurse supervisor's additional responsibilities.

nurse supervisor A nursing position with more responsibilities and requiring more experience than a staff nurse.

Table 5.3	*Employment Settings and Salaries for Nurses*			
	LPNs		**RNs**	
Setting	**% Employed**	**Avg Salary**	**% Employed**	**Avg Salary**
Hospital	20	$42,330	61	$67,210
Office	12	39,930	7	58,420
LTC	38	44,500	7	58,830
Home health	11	45,370	6	62,090

Source: Bureau of Labor Statistics, U.S. Department of Labor. 2014–15. *Occupational outlook handbook, Licensed practical nurses* and *Registered nurses*.

Medical Offices

Medical offices include all the physician offices and clinics where patients receive ambulatory primary care services. In those offices, nurses prepare patients for the health examination and assist with the exam. They also maintain patient records. Nurses perform many of the diagnostic tests once done by physicians and provide clinical care for monitoring patients with chronic disease.

Medical offices also include a number of services that used to be performed only in inpatient hospital settings. More sophisticated procedures, especially outpatient surgery, are now performed in medical offices and surgicenters. Here the nurse may also assist with the surgical procedure and administer medications and injections.

Long-Term Care and Home Health

Both long-term care and home health are providing increased opportunities for nurses. Because of the aging of the population, there is increased demand for long-term care services, especially to care for those with Alzheimer's or as a consequence of stroke or head injuries. Technological advances have made it possible for many complex procedures to be performed in the home, which has increased opportunities in that setting.

In the long-term care facility, the RN usually has an administrative or supervisory role. LPNs perform direct patient care tasks (Bureau of Labor Statistics, RNs and LPNs 2014–15). Home health care offers the opportunity to work independently. Both settings expect to see an increased demand for aides. Part of this is related to the growth in these settings, but part of it is because of high turnover among the aides. Their pay is low, with little opportunity to move up, and the job has high physical and emotional demands.

Public Health

As the health care industry shifts from an emphasis on treating disease to an emphasis on preventing disease, the industry has paid more attention to the public health setting. Nurses in this setting provide primary care services to the community, including immunizations, screenings, and pediatric care. They also play an important role as educators, instructing the community about health issues, disease prevention, and nutrition. Public health nurses must have at least a bachelor's degree.

Other Opportunities

Nurses who choose not to provide care directly to patients can find employment on the business side of health care. Many companies that provide home health and chronic care services employ nurses in management positions. In those positions, nurses perform the managerial roles of planning and development, marketing, and quality assurance. Their nursing experience provides the companies they work for with valuable insights. Nurses who decide to take this employment direction usually return to school for graduate-level management education.

Another area of employment is in education. Nursing faculty are in high demand. Those with a master's or a doctorate administer educational programs, as well as teach.

Issues in Health Care Delivery

As discussed earlier in this text, the health care industry faces challenges to improve access, maintain quality, and control costs. These are serious concerns for everyone employed in the health care industry. The same supply and demand concerns that affect the overall economy are present in the health care industry.

There is concern that there is an insufficient supply of health care providers of all types. Part of the problem lies in attracting applicants, but this chapter has demonstrated that both medical and nursing schools have more applicants than they can admit. To expand educational opportunities is a multiyear endeavor, requiring the construction and equipping of expensive facilities and an increase in the number of professionals who are willing to become faculty, often at lower salaries than what they can earn as practitioners. Rigorous educational and licensure requirements encourage quality, but restrict people from entering the profession.

To increase the supply of physicians, some states have developed incentive programs where they will pay for medical school if the physician promises to practice in an underserved area. As well as calling for medical schools to control costs, the AMA also supports an income tax deduction for the interest on medical school loans. States have also looked for ways to fund initiatives that would increase the number of nurses.

Another part of the problem lies in retaining people in health care professions. **Burnout** is common in professions that demand a great deal of empathy from their practitioners. Burnout is generally caused by stress and overwork, both of which are common in health settings that are understaffed. Other serious concerns included back injuries, **needlestick injuries, latex allergies**, and physical and verbal abuse. The wide variance in compensation between various clinical providers can be another source of dissatisfaction that causes people to change professions.

Matching the supply of clinical providers to the demand for their services also causes gaps. Cost pressures in particular have led to staffing with less expensive professionals. The more expensive RN is replaced with the less expensive LPN or NA, or the patient is seen by a nurse practitioner instead of a primary care physician. Depending on the setting, this can raise questions about the quality of services provided to a patient.

The way services are billed and reimbursed also influences demand. Nursing care is not billed separately (it is part of the daily fee for hospitals, for example). Insurance may cover visits to one type of care provider, but not to another. Concerns about quality of care have influenced legislators and accrediting agencies to look closely at staffing levels, which then alter the demand for certain kinds of clinical providers.

burnout
A psychological condition in which a person loses the ability to care and becomes apathetic. Stress and overwork are thought to cause burnout.

needlestick injuries
Health practitioners can be injured and exposed to disease if they are inadvertently stuck by a needle.

latex allergies Many medical practitioners and patients are allergic to latex, which is the most commonly found material in gloves used in medical procedures.

Summary

The ways in which physicians and nurses deliver patient care are described. Physicians, whether MDs or DOs, see patients to diagnose and treat injuries and illness. Physicians are primary care providers or may choose an area of specialty. Most physicians work in some form of office-based practice. In addition to the required education and training, physicians must be licensed by the state to practice medicine. Physicians may describe themselves as "board certified" if they pass the residency and examination requirements of the American Board of Medical Specialties.

The nurses' role in the health care team is "taking care of people." The actual day-to-day tasks are determined by the nurse's employment setting and the licensure. Nursing care is provided by nursing aides, licensed practical nurses (LPNs), registered nurses (RNs), and advanced practice nurses. The State Board of Nursing specifies what educational and clinical requirements are necessary to obtain a license in that state; nurses must be licensed to practice. Nurses work in hospitals, medical offices, and long-term and home health care settings.

The supply of and demand for health care providers influence physicians and nurses. Access to care and quality while still controlling costs are concerns facing physicians and nurses.

Questions for Review

1. What tasks does the physician perform to provide health care services?
2. Describe the specialties of family practitioners, pediatricians, and surgeons.
3. Explain the difference between licensure and certification.
4. What are some of the differences between LPNs and RNs?
5. Describe one type of advanced practice nurse.
6. What is a Nurse Practice Act?

Questions for Discussion

1. As a patient, do the demographic characteristics of a health care provider (gender, race, age) make any difference to you? Should part of providers' education include more diversity training?
2. Many people believe that health care wouldn't be so expensive if doctors didn't get paid so much. What do you think about physicians' earnings and compensation?
3. Suggest ways that nurses can influence public opinion about the scope of the health care services they provide.
4. One argument used for allowing nurse practitioners more independent responsibility is that they are cost-effective providers of care. Do you believe this is a good strategy to improve access to care? Should advanced practice nurses be able to practice without supervision?
5. Interview a physician you know. Does he or she face any of the same concerns as Dr. Hunter (in the chapter profile) does?

Chapter References

American Association of Nurse Anesthetists (www.aana.com).

American Association of Nurse Practitioners (www.aanp.org).

American Medical Association Insurance. 2014. *2014 Work/life profiles of today's U.S. physician.* Chicago, IL: Author.

Association of American Medical Colleges (AAMC). 2014. *AAMC Facts: Applicants, matriculants, enrollment, graduates, MD/PhD, and residency applicants data.* Table 8.

_____. October 2014. *Medical student education: Debt, costs, and loan repayment fact card.*

_____. 2014. *Diversity in the physician workforce: Facts and figures 2014.*

_____. May 2014. *Graduation rates and attrition factors for U.S. medical school students. Analysis in brief.*

Beck, A. 2004. The Flexner report and the standardization of American medical education. *Journal of the American Medical Association* 291: 2139–40.

Blais, K., and J. Hayes. 2015. *Professional nursing practice.* 7th ed. Hoboken, NJ: Prentice Hall.

Bulechek, G., H. Butcher, J. Dochteman, and C. Wagner. 2012. *Nursing interventions classification (NIC).* 6th ed. St. Louis, MO: C. V. Mosby.

Bureau of Labor Statistics, Department of Labor. 2014–15. *Occupational outlook handbook.* Licensed practical and licensed vocational nurses. Available at www.bls.gov/ooh.

_____. Nursing assistants and orderlies.

_____. Physicians and surgeons.

_____. Registered nurses.

Harrington, N., and C. Terry. 2012. *LPN to RN transitions.* 4th ed. Philadelphia: Lippincott, Williams & Wilkins.

Health Resources and Services Administration (HRSA), U.S. Department of Health and Human Services. 2013. *The U.S. nursing workforce: Trends in supply and education.* Available at http://bhpr.hrsa.gov/healthworkforce/supplydemand/nursing/nursingworkforce/nursingworkforcefullreport.pdf.

Hill, S., and H. Howlett. 2012. *Success in practical/vocational nursing: From student to leader.* 7th ed. Philadelphia: W. B. Saunders.

Joel, L., and L. Kelly. 2001. *The nursing experience: Trends, challenges, and transitions.* 4th ed. New York: McGraw-Hill.

Moorhead, S., M. Johnson, M. Maas, and E. Swanson. 2012. *Nursing outcomes classification (NOC).* 5th ed. St. Louis, MO: C. V. Mosby.

National Board of Medical Examiners (www.nbme.org).

Society for Hospital Medicine (SHM). 2014. *State of hospital medicine report.* Philadelphia: Author.

Sorrentino, S., and L. Remmert. 2013. *Mosby's essentials for nursing assistants.* 5th ed. St. Louis, MO: C. V. Mosby.

For Additional Information

Accreditation Council for Graduate Medical Education (www.acgme.org).

American Association of Colleges of Nursing (www.aacn.nche.edu).

American Board of Medical Specialties (www.abms.org).

American Nurses Association (www.nursingworld.org).

National Council of State Boards of Nursing (www.ncsbn.org).

National League for Nursing (www.nln.org).

Other Clinical and Non-Clinical Health Care Providers

Learning Objectives

After reading this chapter, you should be able to:

1. Identify the role of physician assistants, medical assistants, and surgical technologists in hospital and office visits.
2. List the providers of diagnostic testing.
3. Identify the providers of therapeutic services.
4. Describe the role of health care professionals in emergency care situations.
5. Identify the role of dentists, optometrists, chiropractors, podiatrists, and dietitians/nutritionists in the health care system.
6. Define health administration.
7. Identify the role of health information managers and technicians.
8. Describe the role of professional billing and coding in the service delivery process.

Speech-Language Pathologist

Julie Pierce went to college thinking she wanted to be a nurse, but she quickly discovered nursing wasn't her field. A friend in speech pathology urged her to talk to the professors in that department. Julie did, took the introductory courses, and fell in love with the field of speech-language pathology. She obtained her bachelor's degree in communication disorders and her master's in speech-language pathology. After a year of clinical practice under the direction of a licensed speech pathologist, Julie obtained her licensure. The rest, as they say, is history.

Julie is employed by a rural school district in Arkansas as the speech-language pathologist. She sees 20 to 25 children each day, usually in groups of three or four. Her patients range in age from preschool to high school. In the morning, she works with the younger children. Most of what she does is articulation therapy, the actual producing of a specific sound. She starts with the sound, moves on to the word, the phrase, the sentence, and then conversation. When the child can successfully produce the sound in all of those settings, then the child graduates. Younger children are identified by their teachers and then tested by Julie to see if her services are needed. She also spends about an hour a day in the resource room doing overall lessons. Julie also does some language therapy, which focuses on the process of communication. She might work on speech or phrases or on the broader context of appropriate social behavior. Julie's services are free for the student; her salary is paid by the school district. An Individual Education Plan (IEP) is prepared for each student, and conferences are held regularly with parents to inform them of their child's progress.

Introduction

If the physician's role focuses on diagnostics and the nurse's role focuses on caregiving, what roles are played by the other 200-plus health care occupations? This chapter cannot cover every health occupation, but it addresses some office-based occupations, diagnostic and laboratory services, and therapeutic services. In holistic patient care, the health care team encompasses many other clinical and non-clinical health care providers. Patients generally do not encounter many of these other health care professionals until they have seen their primary care physician, been admitted to the hospital, or had a medical emergency. Patients encounter many other health care professionals as part of a total health care program. This chapter also introduces the many non-clinical occupations available in the health care setting. Non-clinical employees use their skills and training to keep the businesses operating so that clinical employees can deliver patient care. Many of these forms of employment can be found in any business, but some, such as health information manager or coding specialist, are only found in health care. Figure 6.1 presents a list of the other clinical professionals covered in the chapter.

Speech pathologists generally work with children or with adults. During their graduate training, students work with both groups of patients. They even experience many of the same tests their patients do. For example, to test a patient's ability to swallow, a moving video is taken of the patient swallowing a barium solution. "It was nasty," said Julie, "but now you know what it's like for the patient." Generally, there are more successes working with children. "Their bodies are amazing at regenerating," says Julie. Adult patients often need therapy as a result of traumatic brain injury or dementia. Although there are occasional gains, the work can be frustrating because the patient's overall condition is likely to deteriorate.

Julie says she prefers working with children because "I'd rather be thrown up on by a child than an adult!" She cautions that speech-language pathology is not a field for "the faint of heart. You're knee-deep in the mouth. I've been thrown up on, spat on, and even choked." What she loves, however, is helping people communicate. "It's wonderful when they grasp an idea. You can see the light come on."

Like many professionals in health care, Julie finds the paperwork and bureaucracy the most difficult part of her job. "It's hard to see a child slip through the cracks because the funding isn't there." She notes that adults face some of the same funding challenges. Speech therapy and physical therapy are grouped together by Medicare without sufficient funding to obtain both. "A stroke victim in a nursing home has to make a choice between walking and talking. That's sad."

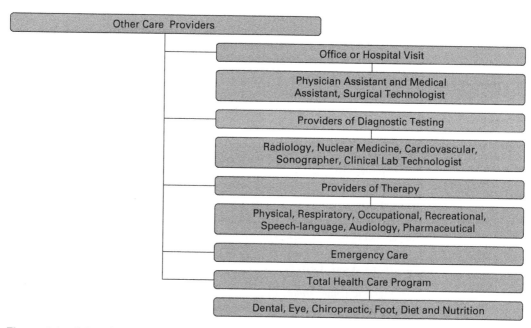

Figure 6.1 Other Care Providers

Office or Hospital Visit

In conjunction with an office or hospital visit, a patient comes into contact with other health care providers in addition to physicians and nurses. These include physician assistants and medical assistants in the office setting and surgical technologists in the surgical setting.

Physician Assistants

There were approximately 86,700 practicing physician assistants (PAs) as of 2012 (Bureau of Labor Statistics, Physician Assistant 2014–15). Working under the supervision of a physician, the PA provides health care services to patients. According to the American Academy of Physician Assistants, this can include taking medical histories, examining patients, ordering tests and X-rays, diagnosing, and prescribing medications (www.aapa.org). In 2012, 23 percent of PAs worked in hospitals, and another 58 percent worked with group practice physicians; the majority are employed full-time.

In all 50 states, the District of Columbia, Guam, and the Commonwealth of the Northern Mariana Islands, PAs are allowed to prescribe medications (www.aapa.org). PAs are particularly in demand in rural and inner-city areas where it has been difficult to attract physicians. In these areas, the PA may be the principal care provider, reporting to the physician on the 1 or 2 days per week that the physician is present.

By state law, PAs must complete an accredited, formal education program; in 2012, 170 programs nationwide provided physician assistant programs (Bureau of Labor Statistics, Physician Assistant 2014–15). The majority of PAs hold a bachelor's degree, although PAs are employable with an associate's degree. Master's degrees in PA are available from most programs. With additional clinical hours, PAs can specialize in pediatrics, orthopedics, or surgery.

In addition to formal education, all states require that PAs pass the Physician Assistants National Certifying Examination (PANCE). Every 2 years, the PA must complete 100 hours of continuing medical education, and beginning in 2014, the PA must be recertified every 10 years.

The Bureau of Labor Statistics indicates that median earnings for PAs were about $93,930 in 2012 (Bureau of Labor Statistics, Physician Assistant 2014–15). As with other health care professions, earnings vary considerably depending on location, specialty, and experience.

Because PAs represent a cost-effective way to provide routine health services, demand is expected to grow by at least 38 percent between 2012 and 2022. Movements to restrict the number of hours physician residents may work and a reduction in the number of residents in teaching hospitals will also increase the need for more PAs.

Medical Assistants

Although the name *medical assistant* sounds very similar to physician assistant, the role of the medical assistant (MA) is quite different. The MA provides administrative and clerical services to the physician. These can include working with patient records, scheduling appointments (including hospital admission and laboratory services), insurance forms, and billing. The MA may also provide limited clinical services to patients. Depending on state law and the size and type of medical practice, an MA's clinical duties might include taking medical histories and vital signs and assisting the physician during the examination of a patient. The MA may also collect and prepare laboratory specimens and perform lab tests (www.aama-ntl.org).

Most MAs have completed either a 1- or 2-year program of college study, resulting in a certificate or associate's degree, respectively. Although there is no licensure requirement for MAs, employers prefer applicants who have passed a national certification examination.

The Bureau of Labor Statistics indicates that there were approximately 569,800 people employed as MAs in 2012, with median earnings of $29,370 (Bureau of Labor Statistics, Medical Assistant 2014–15). According to the American Association of Medical Assistants (2014), 94 percent work in physicians' offices, with more than half in specialty practices. MA is one of the fastest-growing occupations because of the increase in the number of health care facilities that rely on a high proportion of support personnel.

Surgical Technologists

The patient who requires a surgical procedure, whether performed on an inpatient basis in the hospital or on an outpatient basis in an office, will encounter surgical technologists. They assist the surgical team by preparing patients, preparing surgical instruments and equipment, passing instruments and supplies during surgery, transferring patients after surgery, and cleaning and restocking the operating room. The majority of the 98,500 surgical technologists employed in 2012 worked in hospital operating and delivery rooms. The annual median earnings were $41,790, according to the Department of Labor (Bureau of Labor Statistics, Surgical Technologists 2014–15).

Formal education is acquired in programs lasting from 9 to 24 months. Depending on the length of the program, the surgical technologist earns a certificate or associate's degree. Licensure is not required, but most employers prefer professionally certified technologists. Depending on the certifying organization, certification is renewed through continuing education or reexamination.

Providers of Diagnostic Testing

Physicians frequently order a variety of **diagnostic tests** to provide them with the data to make a diagnosis. **Technologists** and **technicians** provide these services. The difference in the two titles represents the difference in amount of education and training. The most common form of training is a 2-year associate's degree, although some fields require a bachelor's degree. Many health care professionals cross-train by receiving a 1-year certificate. Growth is predicted in these fields because of the health care needs of an aging population. Technologists and technicians are found in hospitals, physicians' offices, and diagnostic imaging centers. Data concerning these career fields are presented in Table 6.1.

diagnostic tests tests ordered by a physician to provide information that assists in making a diagnosis.

technologist A professional who performs testing services. A technologist usually has more training than a technician.

technician A person who performs the routine tasks in a laboratory setting.

Table 6.1	*Diagnostic Testing Careers 2012*			
Position	**No. of Jobs**	**Annual Earnings**	**Education**	**License**
Radiology	229,300	$55,910	Associate's	Y (38 states)
Nuclear medicine	20,900	$70,180	Associate's	Y (25 states)
Cardiology	51,600	$52,070	Associate's	N
Sonography	58,800	$65,860	Associate's	N
Clinical lab	164,300	$57,580	Bachelor's	Varies

Source: Bureau of Labor Statistics, U.S. Department of Labor, *Occupational Outlook Handbook,* 2014–15.

Medical Imaging Technologists and Technicians

imaging technology
a broad term referring to the many forms of technology that allow an image of the patient's body to be produced.

Radiology is the field of medicine that utilizes X-ray and other **imaging technology** to diagnose medical problems. The technologists and technicians in this field (often called diagnostic imaging technicians or radiographers) work with the physician to take X-rays or other tests. A CT technologist uses tomography scanners to produce cross-sectional images of the patients' bodies. Magnetic resonance imaging (MRI) technologists use magnets and radio waves instead of radiation to produce images (www.asrt.org). More than half of all jobs are in the hospital setting. Since 1981 when Congress passed the Consumer–Patient Radiation Health and Safety Act, federal voluntary standards have protected both patients and practitioners from excessive exposure to radiation.

Nuclear Medicine Technologists

Nuclear medicine uses radioactive drugs to diagnose and treat disease. The nuclear medicine technologist administers the radiopharmaceutical and operates the imaging equipment that traces the drug in the patient's body. Almost 65 percent of technologists work in hospitals (Bureau of Labor Statistics, Nuclear Medicine Technologists 2014–15). All technologists must comply with the federal standards regarding the administration of radioactive drugs and the operation of radiation detection equipment.

Cardiovascular Technologists and Technicians

As implied by the name *cardiovascular,* these technologists and technicians specialize in the heart and its peripheral blood vessels. The majority work in hospitals, most commonly in the cardiology department. Technologists specialize in invasive cardiology, echocardiography, or vascular technology (Bureau of Labor Statistics, Diagnostic Medical Sonographer and Cardiovascular Technologists and Technicians 2014–15).

Cardiovascular technologists, those specializing in invasive cardiology, assist with cardiac catheterizations and balloon angioplasty. They may also monitor patients during open-heart surgery. Noninvasive tests involve the use of ultrasound instrumentation. Vascular technologists or sonographers listen to the arteries to diagnose circulation disorders. Echocardiographers, or cardiac sonographers, use ultrasound to examine the chambers, valves, and vessels of the heart.

Cardiovascular technicians receive 8 to 16 weeks of on-the-job training to take basic electrocardiographs (EKGs). Those with advanced training can perform Holter monitoring and stress testing.

Diagnostic Medical Sonographer

Ultrasonography uses sound waves to generate an image to assess and diagnose various medical conditions. The best known use is in obstetrics, where an ultrasound is used to examine the growth and health of the fetus. However, a number of other medical specialties utilize ultrasound technology. Abdominal sonographers scan the abdominal cavity to assess the gallbladder, bile ducts, kidneys, liver, pancreas, and spleen. Neurosonographers focus on the nervous system, including the brain. Ophthalmologic sonographers study the eyes (www.sdms.org). Approximately 60 percent of sonographers are employed by hospitals (Bureau of Labor Statistics, Diagnostic Medical Sonographer and Cardiovascular Technologists and Technicians 2014–15).

Medical Laboratory Specialists

Laboratory testing of patients' body fluids, tissues, and cells plays an integral role in the diagnosis and treatment of disease. Medical laboratory specialists (formerly called clinical laboratory technologists or medical technologists) perform a variety of complex tests on the samples they receive. If they work for a larger lab, they may specialize in the type of testing they do. Clinical chemistry technologists analyze the chemical and hormonal contents of body fluids; microbiology technologists examine bacteria and other microorganisms; immunohematology technologists examine blood; immunology technologists focus on the human immune system; cytotechnologists examine cells for signs of cancer; and molecular biology technologists perform genetic tests (Bureau of Labor Statistics, Medical and Clinical Laboratory Technologists and Technicians 2014–15).

Medical technicians or clinical laboratory technicians perform less complex testing than technologists. Consequently the median annual salary of the 161,500 technicians is lower, about $37,240 in 2012. Technicians also have less education, usually an associate's degree. Two areas of specialization for technicians include **histology** technicians, who prepare tissue samples for pathologists, and **phlebotomists**, who collect blood samples.

Some states require that lab personnel be licensed or registered. Advanced education is required to direct or manage a laboratory. Professional certification, although voluntary, is usually a job requirement.

histology the study of body tissues.

phlebotomist A health care professional who collects blood samples.

Therapy Providers

therapy Remedial
treatment of a disorder.

Part of the physician's treatment may be to order **therapy**. Depending on the patient's medical problems, the patient might need the services of a physical, respiratory, occupational, or recreational therapist. They might also need to work with a speech-language pathologist or audiologist. Therapists may work with assistants and aides. They must be properly supervised, and only a specific set of duties may be delegated to them. Table 6.2 presents data concerning these fields.

Physical Therapy

Physical therapists (PTs) help patients restore mobility and manage pain by implementing a treatment plan that utilizes exercise, massage, and other therapies. About two-thirds of PTs are employed by hospitals or in a PT practice. About 25 percent work part-time. Nursing homes, rehabilitation centers, and home health agencies also employ PTs (www.apta.org).

Working under the supervision of the PT, the physical therapy assistant implements treatment plans and reports the outcomes to the PT. Physical therapy aides perform routine support tasks under the PT's supervision.

Respiratory Therapy

Respiratory therapists treat patients with breathing disorders. More than 80 percent work in hospitals in respiratory care, anesthesiology, or pulmonary medicine departments. Entry-level positions often require that the therapist be

Table 6.2	*Therapy Careers 2012*			
Position	**No. of Jobs**	**Annual Earnings**	**Education**	**License**
Physical therapist	204,200	$79,860	Doctorate	Y
PT assistant	71,400	$52,160	Associate's	Y
PT aide	50,000	$23,880	OJT	N
Respiratory therapist	119,300	$55,870	Associate's	Y (49 states)
Occupational therapist	113,200	$75,400	Master's	Y
OT assistant	30,300	$53,240	Associate's	N
OT aide	8,400	$26,850	OJT	N
Recreational therapist	19,800	$42,280	Bachelor's	N
Speech-language pathologist	134,100	$69,870	Master's	Y (47 states)
Audiologist	13,000	$69,720	Doctorate	Y

OJT, on-the-job training.
Source: Bureau of Labor Statistics, U.S. Department of Labor, *Occupational Outlook Handbook,* 2014–15.

certified (certified respiratory therapist); supervisory positions or therapists in intensive care are usually registered (registered respiratory therapist). Although certification or registration is voluntary, the exam is usually a required component of licensure (www.aarc.org).

Occupational Therapy

Occupational therapists (OTs) focus on improving patients' ability to perform daily living and work skills. Occupational therapists may work in hospitals, schools, mental health centers, or rehabilitation centers (www.aota.org).

OT assistants help with activities and exercises in the treatment plan developed by the occupational therapist. OT aides provide treatment support services and perform clerical tasks.

Recreational Therapy

Recreational therapy includes techniques such as arts and crafts, games, dance, drama, and music to improve the emotional and physical well-being of patients. Therapists work in hospitals and long-term care facilities. Many employers prefer to hire certified therapeutic recreation specialists (CTRSs). This certification requires the bachelor's degree, an examination, and 560 hours of internship (Bureau of Labor Statistics, Recreational Therapist 2014–15). Four states require licensure.

Speech-Language Pathologist and Audiologist

Speech-language pathologists and audiologists are also therapists. Speech-language pathologists diagnose and treat a range of problems: speech, language, cognitive, communication, voice, and swallowing (www.asha.org). Audiologists work with patients with hearing, balance, and related problems (www.audiology.org). More than half of these pathologists and audiologists work in school settings. Health care settings include hospitals and rehabilitation and psychiatric facilities. A small number have independent practices where they do their own diagnostic work or see patients who have been referred by a primary care physician.

Audiologists are required to obtain a doctorate. In addition to the appropriate degree, supervised clinical experience, professional clinical experience, and national examination are required for licensure. Continuing education is usually required to renew the license.

Pharmaceutical Care

Patients who have been to see their primary care physician often don't feel like the visit is complete unless they walk out of that office holding a prescription to be filled. The Food and Drug Administration regulates the pharmaceutical industry and specifies which drugs require a prescription and which can be purchased over-the-counter by the patient/consumer. The pharmacist is forbidden from dispensing any medication without the appropriate prescription.

Table 6.3	*Pharmacy Career Ladder*			
Position	**No. of Jobs**	**Earnings**	**Education**	**License**
Pharmacist	269,900	$106,410/yr	PharmD	Y
Technician	326,300	$13.32/hr	High school/OJT	N

OJT, on-the-job training.
Source: Bureau of Labor Statistics, U.S. Department of Labor, *Occupational Outlook Handbook,* 2014–15.

Depending on state law, only physicians, physician assistants, and nurse practitioners can prescribe. Table 6.3 presents the pharmacy career ladder.

Pharmacists dispense the drugs prescribed by the physician. They also provide information to patients about medications. The majority of pharmacists work in retail pharmacies (43 percent) and hospitals (23 percent; Bureau of Labor Statistics, Pharmacists 2014–15).

While pharmacists hold an advanced degree (PharmD) and must meet state licensing criteria, pharmacy technicians usually have only a high school education and are trained on the job. Many states require certification. Technician job duties include counting tablets, labeling bottles, and other routine tasks. They also verify information, prepare insurance forms, and stock inventory. Questions concerning a prescription are referred to the pharmacist. Three-quarters of technicians work in retail settings, such as pharmacies, general stores, or grocery stores (Bureau of Labor Statistics, Pharmacy Technicians 2014–15).

Emergency Care Providers

Thus far we've seen encounters with health care professionals because the patient has initiated contact with the health care system by visiting the primary care physician. However, in an emergency situation, the patient may enter the system through encounters with a number of emergency care professionals. Emergency care services are locally designed to provide the best care for that community.

In an emergency, EMTs (emergency medical technicians) and paramedics are dispatched to the scene. They provide appropriate medical care on site and transport the patient to the hospital for further care. The precise nature of care depends on the level of training of the EMT.

The National Registry of Emergency Medical Technicians (NREMT) has three levels of service providers: EMT-basic, EMT-intermediate, and paramedic. EMT-basic personnel care for patients at the accident scene and transport by ambulance. EMT-intermediate personnel can administer intravenous fluids, use defibrillators, and use advanced airway techniques and equipment. Paramedics may also administer drugs, interpret EKGs, and use other complex equipment.

Department of Labor data indicate EMTs and paramedics held about 239,100 jobs in 2012 (Bureau of Labor Statistics, Emergency Medical Technicians and Paramedics 2014–15). Although earnings vary considerably as a function of training and geographic location, annual median earnings were about $31,020. Most work for ambulance services. Firefighters often have EMT or paramedic training; they are employed by the municipality.

Training and certification is required to become an EMT and paramedic. The training is a combination of college coursework and clinical and field experience. Paramedics usually obtain an associate's degree. Every state has an agency in charge of emergency services that issues licenses. Most states require that EMTs meet the certification requirements of the National Registry of Emergency Medical Technicians (www.nremt.org).

Total Health Care Program

There are some health care professionals whom patients encounter only if they specifically seek that type of care. No referral is necessary from the primary care physician.

Dental Care

As part of their total health care program, patients must decide who and how they will take care of their teeth. Table 6.4 presents data about the different professionals in dental care.

The dentist is the physician who provides oral health care. Like other physicians, dentists are licensed by the state and may prescribe medications for their patients. Dentists can be general practitioners or specialists. Common areas of specialization include orthodontia, the straightening of teeth; pediatrics, taking care of children's teeth; periodontics, gums and bones; oral surgery, operating on mouth and teeth; and endodontics, root canals. Dentistry has increasingly focused on preventive care, so dentists spend time educating their patients about the proper way to brush and floss their teeth (Bureau of Labor Statistics, Dentists 2014–15).

However, the dentist employs a number of other professionals to provide care. Chief among these are dental hygienists, who do the bulk of health assessment,

Table 6.4	*Dental Care Professionals*			
Position	**No. of Jobs**	**Earnings**	**Education**	**License**
Dentist	146,800	$149,310	DDS	Y
Hygienist	192,800	$70,210	Associate's	Y
Assistant	303,200	$34,500	OJT/college	Y(some)
Lab technician	82,900*	$36,090	OJT/college	N

DDS, doctor of dental surgery; OJT, on-the-job training; *combined number for dental and ophthalmic laboratories.
Source: Bureau of Labor Statistics, U.S. Department of Labor, *Occupational Outlook Handbook,* 2014–15.

X-rays, and teeth cleaning. In some states, hygienists are permitted to perform additional duties related to fillings and surgery. Because many of the routine care tasks previously performed by dentists are now being done by hygienists, the field is expected to grow rapidly (Bureau of Labor Statistics, Dental Hygienists 2014–15).

The dentist's office also employs dental assistants, who perform a combination of patient care, office, and laboratory tasks. Usually the assistant is in charge of the office's infection control procedures. If the assistant is permitted to perform radiological procedures, he or she must pass an exam offered by the Dental Assisting National Board (www.dentalassisting.org).

A large dentist office might have its own laboratory, but it is more common for dental laboratory technicians to work in a commercial dental laboratory. The technician creates all the dental prosthetics such as crowns, bridges, and dentures, as prescribed by the dentist (www.nadl.org).

The American Dental Association has proposed two additional dental care careers. To provide care to underserved communities, the ADA is piloting the Community Dental Health Coordinator. In office settings, the Oral Preventive Assistant provides oral health care education and preventive services for patients (www.ada.org).

Eye Care

As part of their total health care program, patients must decide who and how they will take care of their eyes. More than half of all Americans need corrective eyewear. Disorders such as diabetes or frequent headaches may require specialized vision treatment. Table 6.5 presents data about eye care professionals.

Ophthalmologists are physicians who treat diseases of the eye and perform eye surgery (see Chapter 5). They may also prescribe corrective lenses.

Optometrists provide primary care. Although this includes prescribing corrective lenses, it also includes treating and managing diseases of the visual system, such as cataracts and macular degeneration (www.aoa.org). They are doctors of optometry (ODs). To earn this degree, the optometrist completes a 4-year optometry program, after completing a bachelor's degree or at least 3 years of a pre-optometry program. After passing written and clinical state

Table 6.5	*Eye Care Professionals*			
Position	**No. of Jobs**	**Earnings**	**Education**	**License**
Optometrist	33,110	$97,820	Bachelor's + OD	Y
Optician	67,600	$33,330	Associate's	Y (22 states)
Lab technician	89,900*	$28,590	OJT/college	N

OD, doctor of optometry; OJT, on-the-job training; *combined number for dental and ophthalmic laboratories.
Source: Bureau of Labor Statistics, U.S. Department of Labor, *Occupational Outlook Handbook*, 2014–15.

board examinations, the optometrist is licensed to practice. Continuing education is required to renew the license. About two-thirds of optometrists work in stand-alone offices, but only 11 percent are self-employed (Bureau of Labor Statistics, Optometrists 2014–15).

Dispensing opticians fill the prescriptions written by ophthalmologists and optometrists for the patient's corrective lenses. About 40 percent work directly for the optometrists, and another 32 percent work in retail optical stores (Bureau of Labor Statistics, Opticians 2014–15).

Ophthalmic laboratory technicians actually make the prescription eyeglasses. Contact lenses are usually produced by machine (Bureau of Labor Statistics, Dental and Ophthalmic Laboratory Technicians 2014–15).

Chiropractic Care

Chiropractic has become increasingly accepted as a form of health care, and usually treatment is covered by insurance. The chiropractor's approach to health care is holistic, but the focus is on the spine. Therefore, the primary intervention is manipulation of the spine.

Chiropractors are also known as chiropractic physicians or doctors of chiropractic (DCs). Usually a bachelor's degree and a 4-year chiropractic college course are required to obtain the doctor of chiropractic degree. All states require licensure, which requires formal education and examination, usually through the National Board of Chiropractic Examiners. Continuing education is required to maintain licensure. States vary widely in terms of what they permit chiropractors to do within the scope of their practice. However, all states prohibit chiropractors from prescribing medications and from performing major surgery.

Most chiropractors are in private, solo practice. According to the Department of Labor, in 2012, 44,400 chiropractors had median annual earnings of $66,160 (Bureau of Labor Statistics, Chiropractors 2014–15).

Foot Care

Podiatrists provide specialized care for the foot. There are relatively few podiatrists—about 12,200—and more than half are in solo practice. Average earnings are $113,560. A license is required to practice podiatric medicine. The podiatrist must graduate from one of the nine accredited colleges of podiatric medicine. The program is similar to medical school, where students have clinical rotations in the third and fourth years and complete hospital residency programs after receiving the doctor of podiatric medicine degree (DPM). Podiatrists can also become board certified in orthopedics, surgery, or primary medicine (Bureau of Labor Statistics, Podiatrists 2014–15).

Diet and Nutrition

Dietitians are the food and nutrition experts. Health care practitioners recognize the link between food, fitness, and health. As part of the health care team,

medical nutrition therapy The use of nutrition to support health in a patient.

dietitians provide **medical nutrition therapy** to patients. In addition to direct patient care, dietitians are also employed in wellness programs and public health settings. They often find a role in teaching or research settings, or in food service, whether in a health care setting or in the food industry generally.

In health care, dietitians are frequently employed in hospitals, long-term care facilities, or physicians' clinics. The Department of Labor reports 67,400 people were employed as dietitians in 2012, with a median salary of $55,240 (Bureau of Labor Statistics, Dietitians 2014–15).

Most dietitians and nutritionists hold at least a bachelor's degree, and many obtain a master's degree to progress in the field. The dietetic technician holds an associate's degree. State laws vary regarding licensure and registration.

Health Care Employment in Non-Clinical Positions

In addition to the many clinical providers, patient care is supplemented by the non-clinical providers who keep the delivery systems functioning. These include administrators and managers, health information personnel, and support staff.

Health Administrators and Managers

Health administration is concerned about patient care, but also about profitability and other business issues. Professionals in this industry may be referred to as health administrators, health managers, or health executives, and they hold a variety of job titles. In 2012, there were approximately 315,500 positions in the health care industry, with an average salary of $88,580 (Bureau of Labor Statistics, Medical and Health Services Managers 2014–15). An administrator must understand the basics of management, marketing, and accounting and finance to effectively manage a health care business (Friedman & Kovner 2012). These functions were described in Chapter 2.

Health administration has grown more professional in recent decades. Administrators are often trained in business schools or health administration programs, where they learn business concepts. Some administrators entered their professions as clinical providers and then moved into a management role. Other have a business background but have directed their interest to the health care industry.

Although a bachelor's degree may be sufficient for an entry-level position, most managers have earned a master's degree (www.ache.org). There are three traditional paths: the Master of Business Administration (MBA), the Master of Public Administration (MPA), and the Master of Health Administration (MHA). MBA and MPA programs might include health-related coursework, but only the MHA is completely focused on the health care industry. The American College of Healthcare Executives offers board certifications, which are becoming an industry standard. Some administrators will go on to earn a doctorate, especially if they intend to teach in a university or administer a clinical research setting.

There is some professional tension between the doctors who hold the MD and the doctors who hold the Ph.D.

Careers in Health Information

When used strategically, information technology can assist a health care business to achieve higher level of performance, both of personnel and financially. A variety of professionals manage the information technology needs of health offices. These include the areas of medical records management, privacy officer, risk management, medical coding, corporate compliance, and data analysis and reporting (www.ahima.org). The position of Medical Chief Information Officer has developed as physicians with advanced technical skills develop strategy and policy to meet the organization's IT needs.

Social media is another area of employment growth, as business and technology interact. Websites, Facebook, RSS feeds, podcasts, blogs, and Twitter not only are ways to communicate, but also offer employment opportunities (Thielst 2013). While large companies can afford to have their own IT staff, many smaller offices outsource these functions.

Coding Specialist Increasing computerization of health care recording keeping and the Health Insurance Portability and Accountability Act (HIPAA) requirements for electronic data interchange (EDI) are just two of the factors fueling the growth of coding specialists. The Bureau of Labor Statistics predicts that this field will grow faster than average in the next few years (Bureau of Labor Statistics, Medical Records and Health Information Technician 2014–15).

Based on the documentation provided by the patient's record, coding specialists assign codes, or numbers, to the diagnoses, services, and procedures. That data are used for reimbursement and also to support statistical research. Coding specialists may also be called health information specialists or health insurance specialists. Coders must have a strong background in medical terminology, anatomy, and physiology. Their communication and computer skills (Internet and software) must also be strong. A coder must be able to enter data with accuracy and have the ability to manage details. And of course, the coder must be thoroughly familiar with **CPT** and **ICD-10-CM codes**. After October 1, 2015, ICD-10-CM replaced ICD-9-CM. The transition provided opportunities for those who quickly learned the new codes and can translate from the older version.

In a small practice, a coder may do many types of work tasks. In large practice, a coder's work may be more specialized. For example, one coder may process claims for a single payer such as Medicare. In addition to practice-based employment, a coder has opportunities in other settings. The coder could work for insurance companies, government agencies, private billing practices, or private educators who train medical office employees (Green and Rowell 2014). In 2012, there were 186,300 jobs in the field of medical records and health information technician, with an average salary of approximately $34,160 (Bureau of Labor Statistics, Medical Records and Health Information Technician 2014–15).

Current Procedural Terminology (CPT) A part of the HCPCS used to code procedures and services performed by providers.

ICD-10-CM The abbreviation for the *International Classification of Diseases, 10th Revision, Clinical Modification.* This classification is used to code office visits to process an insurance claim. ICD-10-CM became effective October 1, 2015, and replaced ICD-9-CM.

Coders can obtain professional credentials through two professional organizations: the American Health Information Management Association (AHIMA) and the American Academy of Professional Coders (AAPC). AHIMA offers an entry-level coding credential, the Certified Coding Associate (CCA). When a student demonstrates competency in ICD-10-CM and CPT surgery coding, patient documentation, data integrity/quality, A&P, and pharmacology, he or she can achieve the title of certified coding specialist (CCS). Finally, by demonstrating expertise in multispecialty CPT, ICD-10-CM, and **HCPCS** national (level II) coding, the coder can become a certified coding specialist–physician-based (CCS-P) (www.ahima.org).

Healthcare Common Procedure Coding System (HCPCS) A classification system used to code and process an insurance claim.

AAPC offers credentials that differentiate between patient care settings. For coders in physician practice and clinics, they offer the certified professional coder (CPC) and for coders in outpatient facilities, the certified outpatient coder (COC). AAPC also offers more than 20 specialty coding credentials (www.aapc.com).

Other Support Staff

Transcriptionists and secretaries are among the other support staff necessary to keep health care businesses running. There were about 84,100 jobs as medical transcriptionists in 2012, with an average hourly wage of $16.36 (Bureau of Labor Statistics, Medical Transcriptionist 2014–15). About 34 percent of transcriptionists work in hospitals and another 24 percent in physicians' offices, sometimes combining transcription duties with other tasks such as receptionist. A number of transcriptionists operate home businesses. The skill requirements for transcriptionists evolve as the technology changes (www.ahdionline.org). With the increased ability to send files electronically from anywhere in the globe, there has also been an increase in the use of offshore transcription services, usually to reduce the cost of the service.

As EHR systems become more pervasive, the requirements for medical secretaries have changed. Instead of working for just one person, it is more typical for a secretary to provide support to an entire office or division and to perform a wider range of administrative tasks. There were 516,050 people employed as medical secretaries in 2012, with average earnings of $33,530 (Bureau of Labor Statistics, Secretaries 2014–15).

Issues

As you have seen in this chapter, there are many, many more professions that provide health care services beyond physicians and nurses. In some fields, there are career ladders, so a person can obtain some education and training, go to work in the field, and then get more training and education to advance to a higher position. This practice, although providing opportunities for the individual, creates some concerns about the trade-off between cost-effectiveness and quality. It is more cost-effective to utilize lower level professionals because they are not paid as much. They did not spend as much time training or being educated, so this preparation was also less expensive. The assistant or aide always works under supervision, but some still worry that the quality of care may suffer. Professional associations are also worried that the use of more assistants and aides erodes the professionalism and the earning potential of their specialty.

Related to the concern for cost-effectiveness is the concern about reimbursement. Some services and providers are reimbursed directly; others are not. Changes in reimbursement, especially by Medicare, have a ripple effect to other insurers and then impact the availability of personnel in that specialty.

Summary

In addition to services provided by physicians and nurses, health care services are provided by a wide range of other professionals. In fact, new career fields develop at a fast rate because of patient needs and new technology. In the office setting, the patient encounters physician assistants and medical assistants. The patient encounters surgical technologists in hospital and office-based surgical settings. The physician may order a variety of diagnostic tests such as X-rays, MRIs, and sonograms, as well as testing the patients' body fluids, tissues, and cells. The physician may also order the patient to receive therapy, such as physical or respiratory, and may write a prescription. In emergency care situations, the patient interacts with EMTs and paramedics. As part of a total health plan, the patient may seek assistance for dental, eye, spine, foot, and nutritional care.

In addition to medical professionals, offices, clinics, and hospitals employ many business professionals as well. Health information managers ensure the completeness and accuracy of the health information record, which contains a patient's personal, social, financial, and medical data. Coding and billing specialists ensure that reimbursements process promptly. Health administrators perform business functions such as strategic planning, marketing, and accounting.

Questions for Review

1. What is the difference between the physician assistant and the medical assistant?
2. List three types of technologists and technicians who provide diagnostic testing.
3. What types of services are provided by physical, occupational, and respiratory therapists?
4. What professionals provide care in emergency situations?
5. What services are provided by dentists, optometrists, chiropractors, podiatrists, and dietitians/nutritionists?
6. What activities are performed by the health information manager?
7. List three activities performed by billing and coding specialists.
8. Define health administration.

Questions for Discussion

1. Differentiate among a general practitioner, a nurse practitioner, and a physician assistant. What accounts for the difference in their compensation?
2. Were you surprised at the training levels and compensation of any of these professionals? Why?
3. Do you believe that the use of assistants and aides impacts the quality of care?
4. What factors do you believe drive which professionals receive direct reimbursement?
5. The speech pathologist in the chapter profile noted that Medicare will not pay for all the services a person might need to regain functions. What might be a rationale for such a decision? Can you suggest other ways a health care system could achieve the same goal?
6. Differentiate among the MBA, MPA, and MHA. What accounts for the differences in these degrees?
7. Should clinical and non-clinical professionals be cross-trained? Would this improve either the level of patient care or the efficiency of the business?
8. Is there a profession that was not discussed in this chapter that is of interest to you? If so, do your own search for information. What are the education and training requirements? What can you expect to make?

Chapter References

Academy of Nutrition and Dietetics (www.eatright.org)
Alliance of Cardiovascular Professionals (http://acp-online.org/)
American Academy of Audiology (www.audiology.org)
American Academy of Medical Administrators (www.aama.socious.com)
American Academy of Physician Assistants (www.aapa.org)
American Academy of Professional Coders (www.aapc.com)
American Association for Respiratory Care (www.aarc.org)
American Association of Colleges of Pharmacy (www.aacp.org)
American Association of Medical Assistants (www.aama-ntl.org)
American Association of Pharmacy Technicians (www.pharmacytechnician.com)
American Chiropractic Association (www.acatoday.com)
American College of Healthcare Executives (www.ache.org)
American Dental Assistants Association (www.dentalassistant.org)
American Dental Association (www.ada.org)
American Dental Hygienists' Association (www.adha.org)
American Health Information Management Association (www.ahima.org)
American Occupational Therapy Association (www.aota.org)
American Optometric Association (www.aoa.org)
American Pharmacists Association (www.pharmacist.com)
American Physical Therapy Association (www.apta.org)
American Podiatric Medical Association (www.apma.org)
American Registry of Diagnostic Medical Sonographers (www.ardms.org)
American Society of Echocardiography (www.asecho.org)
American Society of Radiologic Technologists (www.asrt.org)

American Speech-Language-Hearing Association (www.asha.org)

American Therapeutic Recreation Association (www.atra-online.com)

Association for Healthcare Documentation Integrity (www.ahdionline.org)

Association of Surgical Technologists (www.ast.org)

Bureau of Labor Statistics, U.S. Department of Labor. 2014–15. *Occupational Outlook Handbook.* Available at www.bls.gov/ooh/. See sections on Physician Assistant; Medical Assistant; Surgical Technologist; Radiologic and MRI Technologists; Nuclear Medicine Technologists; Diagnostic Medical Sonographer and Cardiovascular Technologists and Technicians; Medical and Clinical Laboratory Technologists and Technicians; Physical Therapists; Physical Therapy Assistants and Aides; Respiratory Therapists; Occupational Therapists; Occupational Therapy Assistants and Aides; Recreational Therapists; Speech-Language Pathologists; Audiologists; Pharmacists; Pharmacy Technicians; Emergency Medical Technicians and Paramedics; Dentist; Dental Hygienists; Dental Assistants; Dental and Ophthalmic Laboratory Technicians; Optometrists; Dispensing Opticians; Chiropractors; Podiatrists; Dietitians; Medical and Health Services Managers; Medical Records and Health Information Technicians; and Medical Transcriptionists.

Friedman, L., and A. Kovner (Eds). 2012. *101 careers in healthcare management.* New York: Springer Publishing Co.

Green, M., and J. Rowell. 2014. *Understanding health insurance: A guide to billing and reimbursement.* 12th ed. New York: Delmar Cengage Learning.

International Chiropractors Association (www.chiropractic.org)

National Association of Chain Drug Stores (www.nacds.org)

National Association of Dental Laboratories (www.nadl.org)

National Association of Emergency Medical Technicians (www.naemt.org)

National Registry of Emergency Medical Technicians (www.nremt.org)

Opticians Association of America (www.oaa.org)

Society for Vascular Ultrasound (www.svunet.org)

Society of Diagnostic Medical Sonography (www.sdms.org)

Thielst, C. 2013. *Social media in healthcare: Connect, communicate, collaborate.* 2nd ed. Chicago, IL: Health Administration Press.

World Chiropractic Alliance (www.worldchiropracticalliance.org)

For Additional Information

Reference any of the websites just listed for additional information about these professions.

HOSP

NEXT

7

Offices, Clinics, and Hospitals

Learning Objectives

After reading this chapter, you should be able to:

1. Describe the ways a health care delivery system can be classified.
2. Describe the contents of a health information record.
3. Distinguish between the types of practice arrangements.
4. List the sources of physicians' revenues.
5. Describe the impact of legal issues and customer relations on practice management.
6. Classify the different types of hospitals.
7. List the role and function of the governing board, medical staff, and hospital administration.
8. Discuss the management, marketing, and finance functions that a hospital administrator must perform.
9. List the various utilization measures that hospital administrators use to evaluate performance.
10. List various measures of health care quality.

The Push Toward Electronic Health Records

The days of jokes about doctors' bad handwriting are coming to an end. Electronic health records (EHR) are replacing paper records in offices and hospitals around the country. In 2013, three-quarters of physicians' offices have some type of EHR; almost 50 percent have a system that meets the federal criteria for a basic system. A basic EHR system has the following capabilities: patient history and demographics, patient problem lists, physician clinical notes, comprehensive list of patients' medications and allergies, computerized orders for prescriptions, and the ability to view laboratory and imaging results electronically.

EHR offers some tremendous advantages. Most practitioners agree that EHR has improved the health of their patients. Errors caused by misreading handwriting or drug interactions can be dramatically reduced, saving both lives and money. The new system can also enhance communications with patients; a physician can link directly to clinical information while seeing the patient. Patients may be able to enter their own health information online and share this information with physicians. Using EHR creates staff efficiencies and patient-flow efficiencies. Because there's no need to pull charts, it may even be possible to add to practice revenues by seeing several more patients per day.

Although the advantages of integrated electronic records are widely recognized, implementing a new system requires effort and money. An effective EHR system combines hardware, software, and tech support and training to achieve the goal: all patient information is available at the point of care. As medical practices make the switch, they need to carefully evaluate the workflows in their practice to determine which system will do the best job for their needs. Critical workflows include billing and accounts receivable, scheduling, in-house messaging, documentation of patient interactions, processing refill requests, reviewing and acting on lab results, and managing external correspondence about patients. One system may not do it all, so the system needs to be compatible with other programs. Sufficient time must be set aside for training. The budget must include funds for annual maintenance fees and future upgrades of software and hardware.

Once an EHR system is in place, offices must be aware of the need for enhanced security for those records. Like any electronically stored data, medical records are vulnerable to hackers. Records that a patient creates with a private vendor are also not covered under physician–patient privacy rules.

Health care providers must implement electronic record systems to be in compliance with federal law. Under the Health Information Technology for Economic and Clinical Health (HITECH) Act of 2009, physicians who adopt EHR may receive incentive payments for "meaningful use." In 2013, 69 percent said they intended to participate in the incentive program, although only 13 percent reported having systems that met all of the criteria. From 2010 to 2013, the ability to send prescriptions to the pharmacy electronically and the abilities to provide warnings of drug interactions or contraindications increased significantly.

Sources: Glandon, G., D. Smaltz, and D. Slovensky. 2013. *Information systems for healthcare management.* 8th ed. Chicago, IL: Health Administration Press; Hsiao, C.-J., and E. Hing. 2014. *Use and characteristics of electronic health record systems among office-based physician practices: United States, 2001–2013.* NCHS data brief, no. 143. Hyattsville, MD: National Center for Health Statistics.

Introduction

In the previous chapters, you have learned about the health care professionals who deliver services to patients as well as other non-clinical employees. In the following chapters, you will learn more about the delivery systems. This chapter focuses on providers' offices, clinics, and hospitals.

There are a number of ways to classify delivery systems and the services that patients receive, and the categories often overlap. Systems can be classified by the physical location in which the services are delivered: office, clinic, hospital, and so on. That is the classification used in this chapter. As you will see, the distinction between which services are provided in an office and which services are provided in a hospital is less obvious than it was even 10 years ago.

The delivery system might also be classified by the patient's condition when the services are received. **Ambulatory care** means that patients are fully mobile—they can bring themselves to the physician's office or to a clinic. **Acute care**, on the other hand, implies a level of urgency. This patient needs access to health care services immediately. Based on the seriousness of the illness, the patient may be admitted to a hospital; the services are then classified as **inpatient care**. Most primary care and even some routine surgery is performed on an **outpatient** basis, meaning there is no need for an overnight stay in a hospital. A third method of classification combines the location of care with a level of care; hence the terms primary, secondary, and tertiary. **Primary care** is defined as basic and routine care that can be delivered in an office or clinic by a primary care provider. **Secondary care** involves routine hospitalization and surgery, and **tertiary care** is complex and specialized care delivered in specific institutional settings. Primary care is the only term that is used with regularity.

Various data can be consulted to understand how many patients are served by each type of delivery system. According to the National Center for Health Statistics, there were over a billion visits to physicians' offices in 2010. Primary care physicians provide almost 55 percent of all preventive care. Most of the visits made to physicians' offices (85.6 percent) were by established patients; 31 percent had made at least one previous visit in the past 12 months. More than half of visits involved a general medical exam, and 75 percent resulted in medication therapy (National Center for Health Statistics 2010). These visits are critical for primary and preventive care—the uninsured have a much lower visit rate, putting them at risk for more serious health issues.

In 2011, 126.7 million visits were made to outpatient departments, and 136 million visits were made to emergency departments. Of the latter, about 23 percent were related to injuries and poisoning, and 11.9 percent resulted in hospital admission (National Center for Health Statistics 2011). Hospital use can be examined by considering discharges; in 2010, there were 35.1 million discharges. Over 51.4 million procedures were performed, and the average hospital stay was 4.8 days.

The U.S. Census Bureau gathers data on various industries every 5 years; the most recent data is from 2012. Comparative data about the business side of

ambulatory care Medical care provided in an office setting to a mobile patient.

acute care Short-term medical care provided to a patient with an immediate need for care.

inpatient care The patient needs care that requires being admitted to the hospital.

outpatient care Also referred to as ambulatory care. The patient does not require admittance to a hospital.

primary care Basic and routine care that can be delivered by a provider in an office or clinic.

secondary care Usually involves routine hospitalization and surgery on a short-term basis.

tertiary care Complex and specialized care delivered in specific institutional settings such as burn treatment.

Table 7.1	*Ambulatory Health Care Services*		
	All Ambulatory Providers	**Physicians' Offices**	**Outpatient Centers**
Establishments (number in 1,000s)	582.7	221.5	34.4
Revenue (in millions)	$825.7	$405.7	$98.9
Employees (number in 1,000s)	6,562	2,269	788.7
Annual payroll (in millions)	$341.4	$178.7	$36.3

Source: U.S. Census Bureau. *2012 Economic Census. Preliminary summary statistics for U.S. Sector 62: Health care and social assistance.* Released 11/25/2014.

ambulatory care are presented in Table 7.1. Along with other segments of the health care industry, this segment is growing. Revenues, payroll, and employees have all increased over the 5-year time period in comparison with 2007 data.

Providers' Offices and Clinics

When the patient visits the office or clinic, he or she interacts with many of the health care professionals whose roles and tasks were described in previous chapters. The patient is seen by the care provider, as well as by various nurses or physician's assistants. The patient may also receive services from an in-house laboratory or imaging center.

The office or clinic is a business as well as a place to obtain health care services. Therefore, the patient will interact with non-clinical or administrative staff. An office manager is responsible for the business side of a professional practice. Depending on the size of the practice, the practice may employ receptionists, filing/record clerks, health information management specialists, coding and billing specialists, accounts receivable clerks, and payroll clerks.

Appointments must be scheduled, patients checked in, their records made ready, information from the current visit added, the records stored appropriately, and further appointments scheduled. All these processes must occur within the privacy guidelines as formulated in Health Insurance Portability and Accountability Act (HIPAA).

In addition to the administrative tasks necessary to handle patients, the office or clinic must be managed like any other business. The business has facilities that must be paid for and maintained. Supplies and equipment, both for the office and for the needs of patients, are acquired and maintained. Appropriate information technology is used and upgraded as necessary. Employees must be hired and trained. Bills, payroll, and taxes need to be paid in a timely fashion. The office manager talks to all the sales reps that are marketing pharmaceuticals, new technology, or other products of interest. The business must be in compliance with the many state and federal laws that apply to all businesses, not just those in the health care industry.

The Health Information Record

As noted in this chapter profile, recording keeping is an important part of health care businesses. When you learned about the payment process earlier in this text, you learned how important billing and coding are to the reimbursement process. The health information record, however, serves a broader purpose than just payment.

Whether it is kept in paper or electronic form, the **health information record** contains two types of patient data. First, it contains the patient's personal, financial, and social data. Second, it also contains the patient's medical data, including descriptions of the patient's history, condition, diagnostic and therapeutic treatment, and the results of treatment (Glandon, Smaltz, and Slovensky 2013). Under the provision of HIPAA, it is mandated to protect the privacy of the entire record, but the second type of data is most sensitive and subject to regulation.

The office's health information manager is responsible for ensuring that the office's records are kept in compliance with state and federal regulations (Glandon, Smaltz, and Slovensky 2013). Many individuals in the office have a role in keeping the record accurate and up-to-date.

The health information record has both clinical and non-clinical uses. On the clinical side, the record provides information for patient care. It also provides data for research activities and public health monitoring, and it can be used for quality improvement within the office. The record is also a legal document of the care a patient has received. Finally, as you learned earlier about the payment process in health care, the health information record provides the information necessary for billing and reimbursement (Green and Rowell 2014).

health information record Contains the patient's personal, financial and social data as well as the medical data. The health information record replaces the term medical record.

Practice Arrangements

In Chapter 2, you learned about the legal forms available to businesses in the United States. The operation of offices and clinics can be arranged in several ways: **solo practice**, group practice, or physician/provider employee. Although the solo practice arrangement has become less common for physicians, it is very typical for dentists and ophthalmologists and for some specialty physicians. Health care providers who are in solo practice are usually legally organized as sole proprietorships.

Group practice allows the individual provider to share facilities, equipment, and personnel. From a personal perspective, it also permits the provider to share the burden of providing care. The **partnership** is the traditional legal structure for a medical group practice. The partnership agreement can be written to handle all the details of how the physician/partners wish to manage the practice. However, each partner remains responsible, or legally liable, for the debts of the partnership. As with any business, these might be ordinary business debts. In a medical practice, they also may be incurred by a malpractice judgment against one of the physician/partners.

Many states now permit professional practices to organize a special type of partnership called a **limited liability partnership** (LLP). The advantage is that each partner's liability is limited to his or her capital contribution. However, the

solo practice A self-employed physician who practices alone.

group practice A group of several physicians who practice as a group.

partnership A form of legal organization of a business involving at least two entities.

limited liability partnership A specific type of partnership arrangement in which a partner's liability is limited to the amount of the capital contribution.

state requires the LLP to carry liability insurance (at least $1 million's worth) to protect against malpractice and other wrongful acts of the partners or the employees of the LLP.

A medical practice can also be organized as a corporation, or a physician may be employed by a corporation. Many states permit the organization of professional corporations (PCs) especially for professionals such as physicians; the PC often must carry individual malpractice insurance. In the case where a physician is employed by a corporation, the physician provides health care services for which the corporation pays him a salary. This is how a health maintenance organization (HMO) works. A group of physicians may also contract their services to a corporation for a fee, as is the case with some managed care organizations (MCOs). In either of these cases, the physician remains personally responsible for his own malpractice, but the employer is not legally responsible.

Physicians and other providers entering this sort of arrangement work under an employment contract that specifies all the details of their employment, including compensation, work obligations, and terminations. It is typical for contracts to also include non-compete and non-solicitation clauses, both of which limit the physician's ability to leave that employer and take patients along or establish their own practice in the same geographic area.

Issues in Practice Management

Physicians and other health care providers are trained to do just that, provide health care services. They are not trained to run businesses. Yet understanding the dynamics of running a successful business is an important part of the total package of primary health care delivery. Managing practice finances, legal compliance, and customer service are all important components.

Practice Finances

The financial health of a medical practice depends on several components. One component is revenue maximization. The other component is cost minimization. Taken together these two components achieve profitability.

The first step is to understand the revenue flows of a practice. As you can see in Table 7.2, physicians' offices receive the bulk of their revenue from patient care, with private insurance and Medicare providing the largest share of payments. At the same time, the office or clinic has expenses in the form of personnel, supplies and equipment, and services such as software, utilities, leases, and liability insurance.

If the provider knows the source of the revenues, then several strategies can be developed to maximize revenues. One strategy is to increase the number of patients seen. This strategy can create ethical dilemmas for practitioners if they feel that an increased patient load is compromising care even as it improves the bottom line. Another strategy is to capture more revenue per patient. Practices can lose money through poor coding and billing practices. They can also lose money because their health plans have low reimbursement or because the practice doesn't keep its fee schedules up-to-date.

Table 7.2	*Revenues and Expenses for Physicians' Offices and Hospitals* (in $ millions)	
	Offices	**Hospitals**
Total Revenue	409.8	947.7
Patient care		
Government	107.8	357.8
Private insurance	185.7	307.6
Patient out-of-pocket	35.1	40.2
Other	57.1	66.4
Non-patient care	21.6	42.8
Total Expenses	375.6	884.2
Personnel	188.5	355.4
Supplies and equip.	39.9	154.8
Services	24.9	67.8
Other	41.3	107.8

Source: U.S. Census Bureau, *2013 Annual Services Report,* Tables 4 and 5. Released 11-19-2014.

At the same time a medical practice works to increase its revenues, it must also understand, control, and reduce its costs. Practices should develop budgets and compare their expenses to national data such as that presented in Table 7.2.

Legal Compliance

All businesses operate in an environment that imposes legal restrictions. In addition to the general legal environment, businesses providing primary health care services also face regulation that is specific to the health care industry. One of the most significant legal areas that impacts all business is **antitrust law**. The federal antitrust laws are designed to prohibit activities that lessen competition in the marketplace. Health care providers are impacted by these laws whenever they purchase or merge practices (Showalter 2014). If two practices merge, no matter how much sense a merger makes from either a business or a patient care perspective, the fact remains that customer choice has been eliminated. The fewer medical practices there are in a geographic area, the more competition is reduced. The remaining practices are moving in the direction of a monopoly, which is prohibited by federal law. Health care providers can also be impacted by antitrust law in the way they set prices for their services. Businesses are not permitted to work together to set prices nor are they allowed to tie the sale of one service to another. Nevertheless, some of the negotiation in managed care contracts approaches this sort of prohibited collusion.

Another area of concern is compliance with regulations such as **HIPAA (Health Insurance Portability and Accountability Act)**. Under HIPAA, patients have the right to access and control their health records. To safeguard protected health information (PHI, or patients' individually identifiable information), health care providers must restrict access to the information and have patients' permission to disclose it. The provider has to give a patient a "Notice of

antitrust law An area of federal law that prohibits monopolization and other activities that lessen competition in the marketplace.

Health Insurance Portability and Accountability Act of 1996 (HIPAA) A federal law that mandates insurance portability and sets up procedures for electronic data exchange.

Privacy Practice" on the patient's first office visit. The signed notice is kept in the patient's file. Patients also needed to sign an authorization/consent form for their PHI to be shared for reasons other than treatment, payment, and health care opportunities. Providers are also responsible for the security of electronic health information, whether that information was stored or transmitted. Realistically, this provision of HIPAA affects every office with a computer, Internet, and e-mail. The Affordable Care Act contains additional provisions regarding the security of EHR.

A final area that has both financial and legal implications for providers is malpractice. **Malpractice** is the act of providing medical services that are below the standard of quality. Health care professionals carry malpractice insurance to protect themselves from financial loss in the event that they lose a malpractice lawsuit. Rising malpractice premiums are a concern for all health care professionals.

malpractice The act of providing professional services that are below the standard of quality for that profession.

Customer Service

In all businesses, improvements in customer service help to retain customers. Generally it is not the actual service, but the customer's perceptions of the service, that matters. Customers, patients in this case, can be surveyed so that the provider can understand what's important to the patient. Once such data are collected, service delivery strategies can be improved to meet patient expectations (Capko 2010).

Effective use of technology can also be used to improve service. More and more practices provide an electronic portal (password protected) so patients can access their own medical history online. Newsletters and blogs help keep patients informed. Appointment reminders can be sent by text.

Hospitals

Like offices and clinics, hospitals are both a physical location for patients to receive care and also a business that must be appropriately managed to ensure that care is high quality and cost effective.

Although hospitals were established in the United States as early as 1752, hospitals as we know them are a recent phenomenon dating from the 1920s (Grinney 1991). Prior to that time, the best medical care was obtained in the home. Even some surgical procedures were conducted in the home.

The first hospitals were charitable institutions created for the poor. At best, the hospital offered food, rest, and shelter. Patients were expected to help with nursing and cleaning and behave in morally appropriate ways. However, those who could afford home care stayed away from hospitals.

The discovery in 1846 that ether could be used as an anesthetic increased the use of surgical procedures, but hospitals were so unsanitary that one out of four patients died. It wasn't until 1865 that modern antiseptic surgery was developed, using carbolic acid to kill germs and heat to sterilize instruments (Grinney 1991).

The advance of modern surgical techniques and the increasing use of technology in medicine changed the way doctors practiced. Now it made sense for the patient to come to the doctor rather than the other way around.

By the 1920s, surgery was the heart of the American hospitals. In addition to charity organizations, there were many for-profit, private institutions. They advertised and offered amenities such as semi-private rooms. Internally, hospitals were staffed by caregivers, including nurses, and administrators who were increasingly professional (Grinney 1991).

The current trend is starting to go the opposite direction, again fueled by technological advances. Many procedures that used to require inpatient care are now performed on an outpatient basis, whether at the hospital, a clinic, or a physician's office. Some care that required specialized nursing can now be done with technology and home health. Still, certain types of care remain the province of the hospital. As discussed earlier, ambulatory patients may come directly to the hospital, or they may be referred by their physician.

Types of Hospitals

According to the government's most recent analysis of the hospital industry, there are more than 6,500 hospitals currently operating in the United States (Census Bureau 2014). Basic operational data are presented in Table 7.3.

Although they share certain characteristics, hospitals are not all the same, either in the kind of business they are or in the kind of services they provide. The primary methods to classify hospitals are by the type of ownership or the type of services provided. However, hospitals may also be classified by size, location, length of stay, or any other measure that provides a meaningful way to compare one hospital to another.

Ownership Hospital ownership is one way to classify hospitals. Hospitals are owned either publicly or privately. **Public hospitals** are actually owned by the federal or state/local government. Federally owned hospitals are often operated for certain groups of patients. The Veterans Administration hospitals are an example. State hospitals are often specialized; for example, many states operate

public hospitals
Hospitals owned by the federal, state, or local government.

Table 7.3	*Hospitals*			
	Establishments (number)	Revenue ($million)	Annual Payroll ($million)	Employees (1000s)
All hospitals	6,552	$860.0	$315.6	5,772
General medical/ Surgical	5,106	806.3	291.8	5,285
Psychiatric/Sub. abuse	571	19.9	10.2	220
Other specialty	869	38.6	15.1	267

Source: U.S. Census Bureau. 2014. *2012 Economic Census. Sector 62: Health care and social assistance.*

psychiatric hospitals. Cities and counties usually operate general hospitals that serve a broad spectrum of that local population. The Emergency Departments of public hospitals located in urban areas frequently provide primary care for the indigent and uninsured.

privately owned hospitals Hospitals owned by nongovernment entities.

Privately owned hospitals can operate on a not-for-profit or a for-profit basis. Formerly called the "voluntary" hospital, the private, not-for-profit hospital is owned by a community association or a nongovernmental entity. **Not-for-profit hospitals** benefit from provisions in state and federal tax regulations that allow them to avoid paying income and property taxes.

not-for-profit hospitals The primary purpose of the hospital is something other than profit.

Private hospitals that operate on a for-profit basis are sometimes known as proprietary hospitals. As with any corporation, the shareholders own the business. Paying customers and cost containment are critical to the financial success of a private hospital. Unlike the not-for-profit, they must pay income and property taxes. They also finance expansion with loans, rather than the tax-exempt bonds that are available to not-for-profits.

general hospitals Hospitals that provide a range of services.

Services Provided Hospitals can also be classified by the types of services they provide for patients. Most hospitals are **general hospitals**—they provide a range of non-specialized services. Specialized services can include some of the federal hospitals noted earlier where services are provided only to certain categories of patients such as veterans. Specialized services also refer to hospitals that treat one type of disease or illness, such as psychiatric hospitals or drug or alcohol addiction treatment.

long-term care The federal health care definition of long-term care is more than 60 days.

Other Categories Other ways to classify hospitals include size, length of stay, and location. Although there is no standard measure of size, the number of beds is one way to indicate hospital size. Small hospitals have fewer than 100 beds, whereas a large hospital might have more than 650 beds. Short-term hospitals refer to average patient stays of less than 30 days; **long-term care** is anything greater than 60 days. Hospitals classified by location usually focus on either rural or urban designations. Both locations face specific challenges in serving their populations. Some rural hospitals were able to convert to Critical Access Hospitals (CAH) under the Medicare Rural Hospital Flexibility Program of the 1997 Balanced Budget Act. This provided additional funds that allowed rural hospitals to upgrade facilities, equipment, and staffing to better serve their communities.

community hospital Non-federal hospital facilities available to the public.

A final descriptor is the **community hospital**. If the facilities are available to the general public, this term includes all nonfederal short-term hospitals whether the services are general or special.

Hospital Organization

Regardless of the way a hospital is classified, hospitals are all structured in a similar fashion. As you can see from Figure 7.1, a typical hospital is organized in three main parts. These are the governing board, the medical staff, and the management team.

ABC Hospital

Figure 7.1 Hospital Organization

The Board of Directors The function of the **governing board** is to set institutional policy and goals. The board is responsible for the financial health of the hospital. Typical board decisions involve the purchase, transfer, or sale of hospital assets, changes in the hospital by-laws, and appointment of new board members. A key decision for the success of the hospital is to hire and evaluate the chief executive officer (CEO).

Who is chosen to be a board member depends on what type of hospital it is. In community hospitals, board members are active businesspeople in their community. This helps them set policy that will serve the needs of the community. Often they serve voluntarily.

Boards meet monthly or quarterly. At their meetings, they review the financial performance of the hospital, hear reports from the committees, and vote on changes in policy. Boards do most of their work through specialized committees. The executive committee interacts with the medical staff. There might also be a finance committee, a buildings and grounds committee, or a public relations committee.

Medical Staff The governing board delegates the responsibility for patient care to the **medical staff**. It is their job to see that patients receive quality care. A physician applies to the hospital for staff membership and clinical privileges. The physician is not an employee of the hospital; he or she is usually in private practice outside the hospital. Membership and privileges simply allow the physician to admit patients to the hospital. In the last two decades, there has been an increased trend toward the use of hospitalists. These physicians have an employment relationship with the hospital; they admit patients that previously would have been admitted by a primary care physician.

The chief of staff leads the medical staff. Usually the chief of staff is elected by the other medical staff according to the medical staff by-laws. The chief of staff interacts with the board and with the management team. The medical staff is organized by their area of medical specialty; each specialty has a chief. For example, the head of cardiology is referred to as the chief of cardiology.

governing board
A group who sets the overall direction for a group or business.

medical staff
Responsibility for quality patient care belongs to the physicians who make up the hospital's medical staff.

The administrative work of the medical staff is carried out by committees. Key committees are the executive committee and the credentials committee. The executive committee governs the activities of the medical staff. The credentials committee focuses on the standards that will be used to grant staff membership and applies those standards to new applicants. Other committees focus on specific hospital departments, such as medical records, or on specific issues, such as quality improvement or utilization.

Management Team The board delegates authority to operate the hospital as a business to the hospital administrator. As in a private business, this person is often called the CEO. As you can see in Figure 7.2, many areas report to the CEO. The CEO delegates the necessary authority to each of the managers of these areas to complete their responsibilities. Unlike the medical staff, all the personnel on the administrative side are employees of the hospital or independent contractors. Required job skills, education, and training can range from low-skill to highly specialized positions. Pay rates vary accordingly.

Patient Services Patients enter the hospital for inpatient, outpatient, or emergency department care. In all cases, the patient's first contact is with the admitting department. Similar to the process in an office or clinic, a health information record is created. The admitting department enters the patient's personal data and insurance information into the hospital computer system. Once the patient has received medical care, a medical record is added to this information. HIPAA regulations regarding the privacy of health information records must be followed. The admitting personnel must have good customer relations skills as well as quick and accurate keyboarding skills.

Nursing Nurses play a vital role in patient care. The director or vice president of nursing is in charge of all the nursing areas; this person might be called the vice president for patient services. In addition to nursing education, the nursing department includes the various areas of patient care such as surgery, clinics,

Figure 7.2 Organization Chart for ABC Hospital Administration

emergency room, and inpatient care. Each area is managed by a nursing supervisor. For more information about the professional training and job duties of the nursing staff, see Chapter 5.

Ancillary Services Key ancillary services include clinical laboratories, radiology, imaging, and anesthesiology. Additional services might include the pharmacy and respiratory or rehabilitative care. One of the difficulties in hospital administration is dual accountability. On the one hand, the ancillary services report to the hospital administrator. However, the physicians are also professionally accountable to the medical staff. Many of the health care professionals who perform these ancillary professional services for the patients and medical staff work as independent contractors. The imaging center, for example, might be located in or adjacent to the hospital facility. It hires and pays its own personnel. The facility contracts with the hospital to perform all its imaging needs.

Support Services Keeping a hospital running requires the services of many people who are not health care professionals. There are three categories of support services: general patient support services, facilities support, and administrative support.

- **General Patient Support:** While the nursing staff looks after the patient's medical needs, other groups assist in providing a pleasant stay. Housekeeping cleans rooms and changes linens. The dietary department plans meals for the patients' special needs as well as running food service for the hospital employees and visitors. Social services, pastoral care, and the **patient advocate** attend to the other needs of patients and their families.

- **Facilities Support:** It takes a lot of effort to keep the physical facility in clean, safe working order. The laundry washes all those sheets, towels, and uniforms. Groundskeepers keep up the outside areas of the hospital. The maintenance department repairs all the mechanical systems like plumbing, electrical, and heat and air. If the hospital has its own parking facilities, these must be maintained and secured. Security is an increased concern for all businesses. A hospital must have security personnel to patrol the grounds and to man certain checkpoints to prevent unauthorized access. In addition, emergency plans are in place to evacuate the hospital in case of fire or other crisis.

- **Administrative Support:** This area is sometimes called materials management. If the hospital needs something, the purchasing department must contact the vendor and authorize the purchase. This is true whether the item is toilet paper or an MRI machine. The receiving department signs off that the item has arrived on site and passes the paperwork to the business office so that the vendor can get paid. All the hospital's supplies must be warehoused until they are needed.

A trend in support services is to consider **outsourcing**. This means that the hospital no longer performs the function with its own personnel. Instead, it

patient advocate
Hospital employee whose role is to take the side of the patient in all discussions and disputes.

outsourcing The process of buying goods or services from another provider rather than performing them by the business.

contracts with a private firm to handle those job duties. Laundry services and medical transcription are two areas that are often outsourced. The hospital can potentially realize large cost savings, particularly because it no longer pays benefits for these employees. However, the decision must be made carefully because the hospital loses some control over performance, and service can be interrupted.

Business Functions Business functions are those departments that take care of the business side of operating the hospital. These include accounting and finance, information services, human resources, and marketing.

Issues Affecting Hospital Administration

Hospital administration is concerned about patient care but also about profitability and other business issues. Furthermore, hospital administrators must be sure that the hospital maintains licensure and accreditation as well as legal compliance. Finally, all hospital employees must be concerned with the quality of care that is provided.

Performance Measurement Standards are used as a way to measure performance. Hospitals can set their own standards, and many use the standards established by The Joint Commission (TJC) as benchmarks. Many organizations have undertaken initiatives such as TQM (Total Quality Management) or Six Sigma to improve their organization's performance (Hopp and Lovejoy 2012).

Close attention to financial flows, such as those presented in Table 7.2, is another mechanism to improve enterprise performance. Many hospitals suffer financial losses because reimbursement schedules don't cover the actual costs of providing care. According to the American Hospital Association, unreimbursed care cost hospitals $45.9 billion in 2012. Hospitals look for new ways to generate revenues such as an outpatient service like a fitness center. Hospitals have also grown increasingly concerned with managing costs.

In addition to monitoring overall expenses and margins, managers use a standard set of **utilization measures** to track and compare the performance of hospitals. Utilization measures include the average daily census, occupancy rates, capacity, average length of stay, inpatient days, and discharges. The average daily census is the average number of beds occupied per day. When that number is divided by the average number of beds, the occupancy rate is obtained. Capacity is the average number of beds available in the facility. Average length of stay is calculated by dividing inpatient days by discharges. Inpatient days is simply a night spent in the hospital, and a discharge is the release of an inpatient from the hospital.

utilization measures
Measures that indicate whether an organization is being used to its full capacity.

Hospital quality can be measured in a number of ways. Quality has traditionally been determined by looking at patient outcomes. This was measured by mortality rates and long-term survival rates. Mortality rates are further broken down by type of procedure. Additional quality measures consider the volume of procedures, staffing levels, rates of infection, error rates, surgical complications, and infection rates. Surveys of patient satisfaction are also conducted; the level of Medicare and Medicaid reimbursement to hospitals is now based in part on survey results from Press Ganey, as mandated by the Affordable Care Act. Data from the best performing hospitals can be used to benchmark performance. Consumers can access hospital quality information at websites such as www.medicare.gov/hospitalcompare/search.html, which allows them to compare outcomes between hospitals.

Licensure, Certification, and Accreditation Every hospital must be licensed to operate by the state in which it is located. Usually it is the department of health that sets the licensure standards. The licensure standards ensure that the physical facility complies with building codes, fire protection, and sanitation. Most states also set minimum requirements for personnel and equipment.

Hospitals can also be certified. This is necessary if the hospital wants to participate in Medicare and Medicaid. To become certified, the facility is inspected by the state health department. If the facility meets the "conditions of participation" developed by the Department of Health and Human Services, then it is certified (http://www.cms.gov/Medicare/Provider-Enrollment-and-Certification/CertificationandComplianc/Hospitals.html).

In addition to licensure and certification, hospitals voluntarily participate in the accreditation standards of TJC (formerly referred to as JCAHO). The facility must pass a site survey visit to determine if it is in compliance with TJC standards. In addition to being a respected measure of quality for the industry, TJC-accredited facilities are eligible for Medicare reimbursement (www.jointcommission.org).

Federal and State Law In addition to complying with the laws mentioned in this chapter, hospitals also must comply with laws that are unique to their operations.

Legislation aimed at improving rural access to hospitals mandated where new facilities could be built. The EMTALA (Emergency Medical Treatment and Labor Act) dictates policy in hospital emergency rooms.

Career Profile: Institutional Development

Have you ever been to a hospital and noticed that some areas have names, such as the Anne Austin Imaging Center or the Wetle Center for Women's Health? The name indicates that a donor has made a gift to the hospital. Development professionals are the ones that focus on making such gifts happen. Development includes events, major gifts programs, foundation grants, capital programs and campaigns, and endowments—a whole spectrum of activities that bring more funds and attention to the hospital or organization. At the entry level, a development assistant might do tasks like processing paperwork to thank donors for donations or soliciting donations for fundraisers. The assistant might organize donor recognition events and post on social media. Most entry-level positions require a bachelor's degree in marketing, public relations, or a related field. Fund-raising experience is a must. To progress in the field, most people obtain a master's degree and certification as a fundraising executive (CRFE). Development professionals can be found in hospitals and all the not-for-profit health-related organizations, such as the American Cancer Society.

Summary

Patient care can be characterized along many different dimensions. Primary care is the basic and routine care that can be delivered in an office or clinic by a primary care provider. Physicians can arrange their practices in several ways; solo, group, and physician employee are the most common. The primary source of physician revenue is patient care, and most is paid by private insurance, Medicare, and the patients themselves. Legal issues include antitrust, HIPAA, and malpractice. Office management requires attention to finances and customer service.

Hospitals are usually classified by the type of ownership or by the services provided. Hospitals may be publicly or privately owned and may be operated on a not-for-profit or for-profit basis. Hospital organization includes the board of directors, the medical staff, and hospital administration. The board sets institutional policy and goals. The medical staff is responsible for patient care. Hospital administrators ensure that the business side of the hospital is operated effectively by reviewing numerous performance measures. Licensure is granted by the state authority. Certification is part of a Health and Human Services process that allows the hospital to receive Medicare and Medicaid payments. Accreditation is a voluntary process that assesses quality. Hospitals also use other methods to ensure quality.

Questions for Review

1. Describe some of the ways care delivered to patients is classified.
2. How are a solo practice and a group practice different?
3. What are the primary sources of physicians' revenues? How is this different for hospitals?
4. What are some of the legal issues facing offices, clinics, and hospitals?
5. Describe one way to classify hospitals.
6. Compare and contrast the role of the medical staff, the governing board, and the administrators in a hospital.

Questions for Discussion

1. What are your major complaints about visiting a physician's office? What suggestions would you make to improve the situation?
2. Is it ethical for a physician to see more patients to increase practice revenues?
3. Research the hospitals in your area. What form of ownership do they have? How many beds and how many employees do they have? How do their financials stack up against national data?
4. Research the use of EHR in your local offices and clinics. What do the users say are the pros and cons of their system? Are these the same as those mentioned in the chapter profile?
5. How do hospitals in your area compare on the quality measures listed in this chapter? Do you believe those measures really get at quality? Are there measures you would use instead?

Chapter References

Capko, J. 2010. *Secrets of the best-run practices.* 2nd ed. Phoenix, MD: Greenbranch Publishing.

Glandon, G., D. Smaltz, and D. Slovensky. 2013. *Information systems for healthcare management.* 8th ed. Chicago, IL: Health Administration Press.

Green, M., and J. Rowell. 2014. *Understanding health insurance: A guide to billing and reimbursement.* 12th ed. New York: Cengage Learning.

Grinney, E. 1991. *The hospital.* New York: Chelsea House.

Hopp, W., and W. Lovejoy. 2012. *Hospital operations: Principles of high efficiency health care.* New York: Pearson.

The Joint Commission (www.jointcommission.org)

National Center for Health Statistics. *National Ambulatory Medical Care Survey: 2011 Emergency Department Summary Tables.* Hyattsville, MD: Author.

National Center for Health Statistics. *National Ambulatory Medical Care Survey: 2011 Outpatient Department Summary Tables.* Hyattsville, MD: Author.

National Center for Health Statistics. *National Ambulatory Medical Care Survey: 2010 Summary Tables.* Hyattsville, MD: Author.

Showalter, J. 2014. *The law of healthcare administration.* 7th ed. Chicago, IL: AUPHA/ HAP Book.

U.S. Census Bureau. *2013 Annual Services Report,* Tables 4 and 5. Released 11-19-2014.

U.S. Census Bureau. *2012 Economic Census. Preliminary summary statistics for U.S. Sector 62: Health care and social assistance.* Released 11-25-2014.

For Additional Information

American Academy of Medical Administrators (www.aama.socious.com)

American College of Healthcare Executives (www.ache.org)

Department of Justice, Health Care Antitrust Division (www.justice.gov/atr/health-care).

Lee, F. 2004. *If Disney ran your hospital.* 6th ed. Bozeman, MT: Second River Healthcare.

Medical Group Management Association (www.mgma.com)

Salamon, J. 2009. *Hospital.* New York: Penguin.

8

Aging in America

Learning Objectives

After reading this chapter, you should be able to:

1. Describe the health care needs of older Americans.

2. Describe the continuum of care for those 65 and older.

3. Explain the various ways this care is provided.

4. Describe how older Americans finance this care.

5. Discuss ethical and political issues inherent in an aging population.

The New Nursing Home Model

Eola Retirement Center is a multilevel retirement center that features independent living apartments, assisted living units, an Alzheimer's unit, extended care unit, intermediate care unit, and skilled care unit, as well as home health and hospice capabilities. It is designed for residents who want to be able to age in place. Located near a moderate-size city, it sits on a 100-acre campus and has 100 independent living units and a 200-bed nursing center. In operation as a nursing center for 50 years, it is owned and operated by a religious organization. The center has 24-hour RN coverage, with a staffing ratio in the nursing center of 1.5 staff members for each resident.

Marge Segura moved into an independent living apartment at Eola a year ago after the death of her husband. She is 78 years old, very active, and involved in the community. Her apartment has a good-sized kitchen and a spare bedroom for visiting children and grandchildren. Her apartment is also equipped with a multitude of aids to help her with her increasing heart disease and arthritis. All the door and cupboard handles are oversized and only require downward pressure, not twisting. She has an emergency call system in case she falls. The bathroom has a walk-in shower with a built-in chair, and the toilets are higher than usual and have a hip replacement seat. Night-lights automatically come on when there is insufficient light, and all the light switches are motion sensors so that if she gets up at night there is no fumbling for a light switch.

As provided by her contract, Marge has one main meal in the dining room. The meals are served restaurant style with a full bar and wine list. She can have a guest for dinner or choose to take more meals in the facility restaurant on a pay-as-you-go basis. There is also a provision to have meals delivered if she cannot get to the dining room. The facility has a health club with an exercise room and a trainer specialized in geriatrics, a swimming pool, and a covered walking trail. There are frequent lectures and concerts at the facility. If at a later time she needs assistance with activities of daily living (ADLs) or instrumental activities of daily living (IADLs), it can be arranged in house. Should she need skilled nursing care, it is also available on site. Marge pays about $3,000 per month for all the services, and she can expect to age in place in this facility.

Contrast this with the nursing home of the past: what a huge difference! Many of these complexes are as large as small towns and have shopping, health care providers, banks, and spas, as well as a full range of rehabilitation and preventative services.

Introduction

Health care for older Americans is and will continue to be one of the fastest-growing sectors of health care and the general economy. The annual spending for Americans over 65 has topped $300 billion since 2010. This sector accounted for 1.5 million jobs in 2012. This is true for several reasons. The first is the aging of the baby boomers. By 2050, there will be an estimated 88 million people over the age of 65, almost double the number of this age group in 2000. Second, during this same period, the number of people over the age of 85 will also double because of the increased life expectancy of the current older population. Finally, the ability to treat diseases that would have resulted in death a few years ago for all ages will add significantly to the population who need health care services. These services include traditional office-based care, in-home care, community-based care, complementary/alternative care, long-term care (in or out of the home), and increasingly, wellness care. Currently the expenditure for personal health care in the United States for Americans 65+ is about 9 percent of GDP, or $800 billion per year, a figure that includes private or out-of-pocket expenses. Health care will be one of the top employers in the United States for many years to come, as the last of the baby boomers has just entered this age group (Harris-Kojetin, Sengupta, Park-Lee, and Valverde 2013).

LTC

Long-term care (LTC) is an umbrella term used to describe a wide variety of services. It accounts for a large proportion (65 percent) of all the spending by government and individuals in this age group, so it will be explored in detail in this chapter. Historically, the term "long-term care" has been used to refer to services and supports to help frail older adults and younger persons with disabilities maintain their daily lives in an institutional setting. The preferred term is currently "long-term services and supports" and includes both health care–related and non–health care–related services. We will continue to use LTC as a shortcut for these services.

The term *LTC* means providing health care services to an individual for more than 90 days. A wide range of care facilities and professionals is involved in LTC. Most of the recipients (80 percent) of LTC assistance receive it in the community. Nursing homes are just one part of LTC, accounting for a small percentage (3.4 percent) of the total care given. LTC also includes hospitals, assisted living and community-based residential facilities, adult day care, respite care, hospice care, rehabilitation centers, mental health facilities (covered in Chapter 9), adult foster homes, children's chronic care facilities, and care provided by family and friends (http://www.aoa.gov/).

Who Needs Long-Term Care?

The simple answer is anyone, child or adult, who has a **chronic condition** requiring assistance for more than 90 days. The U.S. Public Health Service definition is the standard used to determine if the service is in the LTC sector of health care. The period of time a person receives LTC assistance may range from a short time (90–100 days) after a surgery, accident, or chemotherapy to many years in an institutional setting.

chronic condition An illness or injury lasting more than 90 days; a non-acute illness such as asthma.

activities of daily living (ADLs) Basic activities such as mobility, eating, toileting, dressing, and bathing.

instrumental activities of daily living (ADLs) Activities like managing money, telephoning, grocery shopping, personal shopping, using transportation, housekeeping, and managing medications.

The need for LTC is determined by assessing the ability of the person to perform what are called **activities of daily living (ADLs)** and **instrumental activities of daily living (IADLs)**. The ability to perform these activities is assessed according to four categories: (1) totally independent; (2) requiring mechanical assistance only, such as a cane, hearing aid, or special eating utensils; (3) requiring assistance from another person; or (4) unable to do the activity at all. No matter what the disease or condition, if the person can manage most of the ADLs and IADLs alone or with mechanical assistance, he or she does not need LTC. For example, a person with multiple sclerosis may be able to dress himself using assistive devices, be mobile using a motorized wheelchair, transfer from chair to bed and back using a hydraulic lift, and have adaptive bathing, toilet, and cooking facilities. This person is independent and may not need LTC services even though he lives with a considerable degree of disability.

The activities of daily living (ADLs) are bathing, dressing, toileting, transferring (as in from bed to chair), continence control (bowel and bladder control), and eating. About 80 percent of those people receiving LTC assistance in the community demonstrate severe impairments in three to six of these activities. The activity impairments that most frequently cause people to move to a residential care form of LTC are continence control and transferring.

The instrumental activities of daily living (IADLs) are managing money, telephoning, grocery shopping, personal shopping, using transportation, housekeeping, doing chores, and managing medications. Family and friends often provide this care without charge to community residents. The frail elderly people who stay in their homes often have a very good support system in which friends or community volunteer agencies do chores, house and garden maintenance, and shopping and take the person to heath care appointments. Only when this network fails does the person have to either pay for the service in the community or move to a residential facility that provides these and other services.

continuum of care The philosophy that the health care system should facilitate an individual's care from complete independence to dependence.

In an ideal arrangement, the LTC services would be provided by a system that meets the needs of any person who needs assistance in the ADLs or IADLs. A system that would meet not only the physical needs of the person, but would also provide social, mental health, and financial support is envisioned as a **continuum of care**. This ideal would emphasize the wellness or holistic approach rather than the illness or medical model currently used. An individual or family who needs assistance with the continuum of care now may have to interact with as many as 80 different agencies. This is hard enough to do when healthy and very difficult to do when someone is ill or frail.

Who Uses LTC?

People of all ages use LTC services for many reasons. LTC might be necessary because a person is aging, has a disability, or has a chronic disease such as cancer, AIDS, multiple sclerosis, or diabetes. Those recovering from trauma or health events like a stroke or accident may need LTC services. Groups such as children with special needs or veterans may also utilize LTC services. The single largest age group using LTC is 65 years and older. This segment represents about 80 percent of all LTC usage. However, children, young adults, and adults all use the LTC spectrum of care.

Older Americans

The actual data about older Americans rarely matches the stereotypes presented in the media. The typical 65+ older American represents 14 percent of the population, has an income of above $35,000, is a Caucasian woman, and lives alone. Older women outnumber older men by 20 percent. Males are more likely to be married than women; 35 percent of older women are widows.

The financial picture is mixed. Despite media presentations of retired Americans enjoying life on the golf course, 28 percent of this 65+ age group continues to work. The major source of income is Social Security. The median income of women is half of that of men in this age group, reflecting shorter time periods in the workforce at lower wages than men. And older Americans continue to have family responsibilities: in 2013, 536,000 grandparents had responsibility for one or more of their grandchildren.

Due to improvements in health care, among other factors, if you reach 65, you have a good chance of reaching 85. The 85+ age group is projected to triple from 2013 to 2040. However, currently, over 10 percent of this age group is under the poverty line (Administration on Aging 2014).

The primary disease processes that affect this population and cause the need for assistance in the ADLs and IADLs are arthritis, complications of high blood pressure (e.g., stroke, heart disease), diabetes, pulmonary disease, cancers, fractures, and cognitive impairment from Alzheimer's or other dementias.

These demographic trends raise two questions. First, who will be available to care for an aging population? About 31 percent of non-institutionalized older people currently live alone; half of women age 75 and older live alone. This does not necessarily mean that they cannot access help from family and friends, but it is a more vulnerable population.

The second question is how we will fund that care? For a third of Americans older than 65 years, Social Security benefits constitute 87 percent of their income. The median income of older persons in 2013 was $21,225, whereas in 2008 it was $25,503. The median income dropped by over $4,000 in those 5 years, while the actual cost of living and out-of-pocket medical expenses increased. About 4.2 million 65+ people were below the poverty line in 2013, as compared to 3.7 million elderly persons below the poverty level in 2008, a statistically significant increase in poor elderly. Another 2.5 million, or 5.6 percent, of the elderly were classified as "near-poor" (income between the poverty level and 125 percent of this level).

Major sources of income for older people in 2014 were Social Security (86 percent), income from assets (51 percent), private pensions (28 percent), earnings/jobs (28 percent), and government employee pensions (15 percent). It is clear from these statistics that most older persons are on fixed incomes or incomes with modest cost of living increases. As the numbers of elderly continue to rise, the number of people who cannot afford care will also increase (Administration on Aging 2014).

Children

An estimated 17 percent of all children in the United States have a chronic condition that requires some LTC services. School-age children use these services more than the very young.

The nature of the condition varies by age group. Preschool children who require these services often have congenital abnormalities or birth trauma. The most common chronic conditions of the rest of the age groups requiring LTC services are, in order of occurrence, asthma, ADD/ADHD (attention deficit disorder with or without hyperactivity), severe mental disorders such as autism or depression, congenital abnormalities, developmental disabilities, and chronic diseases such as diabetes, cerebral palsy, and AIDS. Many children needing assistance have multiple problems. Families face incredible problems caring for these children ranging from care coordination between many parties to financial issues and family dynamics.

People with Disabilities

Non-institutionalized people with disabilities represent about 19 percent of the American population. This is a very broad term that covers many types of conditions. These conditions include neurological disorders, blindness, paralysis, loss of limbs, chronic illness, mental illness, hearing and speech disorders, and developmental disabilities. The individual may have several conditions and need a wide spectrum of services to continue to live independently.

Veterans

The Department of Veteran Affairs (DVA) is the largest integrated health care system in the world with a $160 billion dollar operating budget. It provides comprehensive health care to inactive members of the military and armed services based on the degree of their service-related disability. Fifty percent of men over the age of 65 are veterans. Since 1930, there has been an organization to oversee the provision of these services. The DVA has three main missions: medical care, training and education, and medical research. It also has the duty to act as backup for the Department of Defense during a war or national emergency for the care of injured military personnel. The military personnel (430,000) from the recent foreign wars and United Nations peacekeeping actions have used this backup service. The DVA also provides shelter for an estimated 50,000 homeless veterans each night, provided 438,398 housing loans, and granted 1,088,000 veterans educational benefits in 2014 (http://www.va.gov/budget/docs/report/2014-VAparPartII.pdf).

In 2014, the DVA treated 6.6 million people; this generated over 800,000 hospital visits and 8.3 million outpatient visits. The DVA has Geriatric Research

Education and Clinical Centers, which provide education and training in gerontology and the clinical care of geriatric patients. Each has a special focus, such as dementia, falls, diabetes, and delivery of health care. It operates 139 medical treatment and rehabilitation facilities and directly employs over 325,000 people.

The DVA also either operates, manages, or contracts with LTC facilities, which care for more than 100,000 veterans a year. The DVA also contracts for LTC with community-based home care, adult day care, inpatient and outpatient hospice care, homemaker/home health care, community residential care, and dementia/Alzheimer's special treatment programs. All parts of the LTC continuum are represented in the DVA system. It is also one of the leading educational and research organizations for chronic and aging care (www1.va.gov/health/).

Who Provides LTC Services?

There are many different providers of LTC. The largest group is unpaid caregivers. Most adults who live in the community rely on family and friends or voluntary organizations such as Meals on Wheels for assistance with ADLs and IADLs. Other community providers include home health care providers, adult day care, hospitals, LTC facilities, hospice, case managers, primary caregivers, and specialized organizations such as the American Lung Association, housing providers, prevention groups, and rehabilitation providers.

Unpaid Caregivers

Most adult people who need help with one or more ADLs or IADLs get that help from a network of family members, friends, church organizations, and voluntary organizations. This help is primarily supplied by women: daughters, daughters-in-laws, neighbors, and women's organizations. This contribution to the health care system in the United States is valued in excess of $450 billion annually (AARP Public Policy Institute 2012).

Over 80 percent of all adults between the ages of 18 and 64 who require LTC receive it from unpaid caregivers. Another 11 percent are served by a combination of paid/unpaid care; only about 9 percent rely entirely on paid care.

The age group over 65 years relies more heavily on a combination of paid and unpaid caregiving. They receive about 41 percent of their care from a combination of unpaid and paid caregivers.

Unpaid caregivers account for about 91 percent of care received. The single largest group of unpaid caregivers is adult children, predominantly daughters. Spouses make up about 24 percent of the total and other relatives about 26 percent. Families then shoulder about 91 percent of the unpaid care, with friends accounting for the remaining 9 percent. These caregivers provide an average of 20 hours a week. Approximately three-fourths of these also work out of the household. One out of every three households (65.7 million people) in America care for family members who need special assistance (AARP 2009).

As the baby boomers move into old age, these proportions will change because there will be fewer adult children to give care. This will become a future policy discussion for financing LTC, which has relied on a huge voluntary base from family. Although there are volunteers and family help in nursing homes and other institutional settings, that help is not calculated in these figures. These figures reflect only community care giving.

Home Health Care

Home health care is the fastest-growing segment of LTC with 2,200 registered facilities providing almost 5 million visits each year (Harris-Kojetin, Sengupta, Park-Lee, and Valverde 2013). Although restrictions on reimbursement from Medicare and other factors have caused the actual number of agencies to decrease, the overall number of clients continues to increase at a rapid rate. This increase will continue into the 2020s because of demographic pressures. The home health industry is roughly divided into two categories: Medicare certified and private. The home health care spectrum also includes hospice care.

Home health care has been a part of the LTC continuum since the 1880s when a routine part of medical care was the visit by nurses in the home to those who could not afford a private nurse. It experienced a decline as the use of hospitals increased for extended stays. But with the decrease in long hospital stays that started in the 1980s, the use of home health visits began to increase dramatically. The increase in high-tech home therapy and the aging population, along with early release from hospital stays, fueled the increase. Since the 1980s, home health care has become a viable option to keep even the frail elderly in their homes as opposed to nursing home placement.

The funding of home health care is accomplished by a combination of federal, state, and personal dollars. Medicare reimbursement for home health visits requires the person to be enrolled in Medicare, be homebound as certified by a physician, and to require skilled nursing care or physical therapy. The person can need only intermittent care, not continuous care. These requirements limit the use of this type of home health care primarily to the 65+ age group.

The second type of home health care is provided by non-Medicare-certified agencies and is financed by out-of-pocket or insurance dollars paid by the patient or family. It is available to a much wider range of clients.

A snapshot of home health clients shows that the majority are 65+ predominantly white, married, and women. Diseases of the circulatory system and heart top the list of diagnoses for home health care clients followed by cancer and injury.

The ability to give high-tech treatments in the home that were once only possible in the hospital has made home health care a valuable part of the treatment of chronic disease. The most frequently given therapies include intravenous (IV) antibiotic therapy, chemotherapy, pain medication, total **parenteral nutrition** and **enteral nutrition**, renal dialysis, and respirator/ventilation therapy.

Staffing for home health agencies includes physicians, registered nurses, nutritionists, clinical pharmacists, social workers, home health aides, speech

parenteral nutrition
Any method of delivering nutrition that is not by mouth, such as by an intravenous line or by a direct tube into the stomach or intestine.

enteral nutrition
Nutrition delivered by a tube to the intestines. Example–nasogastric feeding tube.

pathologists, and physical therapists, as well as managers, coders and billers, and other office staff support. Home health care agencies may also give hospice care and would then add grief counselors and family support to the staffing mix.

Adult Day Care and Respite Care

Adult day care allows clients to receive LTC services in a senior or other center for part of each day. In 2012 there were 4,800 registered adult day care centers, providing 273,000 older Americans with services daily (Harris-Kojetin, Sengupta, Park-Lee, and Valverde 2013). Over half of the clients have significant cognitive impairments, and over 40 percent require assistance with three or more ADLs. These clients live at home and may come to the center for a few days each week or daily. The center may provide transportation services to and from the center as well as nursing, social services, rehabilitation services, meals, counseling, and a comfortable social setting. The average age of the clients is 76, and most clients are women, according to the Urban Institute report.

Respite care for unpaid caregivers is an important function of adult day care centers, allowing the caregivers to have scheduled times in which to do shopping, caring for their own health, and socializing with healthy friends and relatives. Nursing homes may also provide longer-term respite care for spouses and family. This might include caring for a person whose spouse becomes ill or a family that needs a vacation from the 24/7 care needs of a cognitively impaired family member.

Adult day care centers may be stand-alone centers or associated with senior centers, nursing homes, hospitals, or home health agencies. The funding for these centers is primarily from Medicaid funds and out-of-pocket dollars from the families. Other sources are Social Security, DVA, Title III funds, state funding, charitable organizations, and private giving funds.

This segment of LTC is growing because of the aging of America, the increased numbers of young adults with disabling chronic disease, the preference for non-institutionalized care, and the cost savings afforded by this model of community-based care.

Hospitals

Hospitals are increasingly offering different types of LTC. A hospital may coordinate discharge services through a hospital home health agency. Many hospitals now operate a home health agency among the outpatient services provided by the hospital. Hospitals may designate beds as certified skilled nursing beds, so when a patient is discharged the patient can be admitted immediately to the skilled unit for rehabilitation services, ostomy management, or chemotherapy. Many hospitals provide the clinical pharmacy or respiratory care for patients under separate contracts with home health agencies. Hospital social services may do case management for some clients, particularly veterans or those covered under special funding sources. Hospitals are often the source for geriatric and psychiatric geriatric assessments and care services.

Increasingly hospitals have specific LTC services under their umbrella, such as adult day care services, hospice, intermediate and skilled nursing facilities, assisted living, and retirement housing. In a sense, the large multilevel hospitals offer cradle-to-grave services.

Nursing Homes

nursing home An old-fashioned word designating a chronic care facility.

A **nursing home** is defined by the National Center for Health Statistics as a facility with three or more beds that is licensed as a nursing home by its state, certified as a Medicare facility, or a designated nursing care unit of a retirement center to provide nursing or medical care. Nursing homes are a rapidly changing part of the LTC spectrum. In the past, the nursing home was a small, often family-owned provider of 24/7 care for the elderly and clients with mental retardation. Now the reality is a corporate multilevel, multifacility modern system of care that may have more than 1,000 beds.

Almost 1.5 million people live in nursing homes in the United States. Residents primarily are 75 years and older (70 percent), while 15 percent are ages 65–75, and 15 percent are younger than 65. Females account for 68 percent of admissions, and the overwhelming ethnic group is Caucasian (80 percent) with 5 percent Hispanic and 14 percent non-Hispanic Black. The primary reasons for admission to nursing homes are ADL deficiencies in bathing, toileting, dressing, and mobility. Over 45 percent of all nursing home residents are diagnosed with either dementia or depression or both (Harris-Kojetin, Sengupta, Park-Lee, and Valverde 2013).

proprietary Owned by an individual or group of individuals: a for-profit arrangement.

Nursing homes can be classified according to ownership characteristics. **Proprietary** nursing homes are for-profit organizations that may be owned by individuals or corporations or be part of a chain. Not-for-profit nursing homes are institutions usually run by charitable organizations or religious groups. Governmental ownership includes county- and state-run facilities as well as the DVA facilities. In 2012, there were 15,700 registered nursing homes in America; 68 percent are operated on a for-profit model, 25 percent not-for-profit, and 7 percent government.

The four categories of traditional nursing homes are the extended care facility (ECF), intermediate care facility (ICF), intermediate care for the mentally retarded (ICF-MR), and Skilled Nursing Facility (SNF). Each is defined by the type and level of nursing care given. This type of care delivery is essentially a medical model with nurses providing and supervising the ongoing care of the patient. The emphasis is on the physical care of the client. The federal government defines the levels of care for reimbursement and certification by Medicare/Medicaid and other federal/state programs. Each level has criteria that have to be met to be certified. These criteria include the minimum type of care that is given in each level. In the SNF, the client receives types of care that range from ventilator care to medication assessment and intensive rehabilitation programs. The SNF must have a registered nurse on duty at least 8 hours a day. Often there are registered nurses on duty 16 hours a day, with LPN coverage at night. The length of stay in the SNF has changed over the last decade as hospitals discharge patients earlier who still need skilled nursing care; the SNF has become an extension of the hospital. The ICF primarily maintains functional ability, assessing and monitoring medication administration and treating chronic conditions. The ECF is primarily for assisting in critical ADLs like eating and toileting. Many nursing facilities have special units for the cognitively impaired client or special rehabilitation units.

Unlike traditional nursing homes, **assisted living facilities (ALFs) or Residential Care Communities** do not adopt the medical model. Rather they emphasize the social/cognitive care of residents. There are more than 36,000 assisted living facilities in the United States housing 910,000 people. The average age of all assisted living residents is 84. The average female-to-male ratio in assisted living residences is 3.5 women to 1 man (http://www.aarp.org/relationships/caregiving-resource-center).

Each unit is a full living unit; it must have a kitchen (often with microwave, small appliances, and refrigerator) and bath and sleeping quarters separate from a living space. Each apartment has special features to assist with ADLs and is specifically designed to increase the ability to maintain independence. These features include handrails, adaptive shelving and sinks to accommodate wheelchairs or other mobility assist devices, automatic lighting, an intercom help system, and special fixtures. The residents eat at least one meal in a congregate dining area. They may get some assistance with medications and ADLs, but the purpose of the ALF is to allow the individual to remain functional and be able to make choices about independence without the restrictive safety regulations that the ICF must impose to keep licensed.

The annual cost for assisted living is estimated at $43,200. However, costs vary widely depending on the level of accommodations, geographic location, and range of services provided (Genworth 2015). In some states, these facilities may receive Medicaid funding with a federal waiver.

Independent living is just that, an apartment specially adapted so that the resident can live without assistance. However, these facilities include a very important restriction: age (usually 60 or 62). Independent living units are often part of a larger multilevel facility. They may actually have all the adaptive features of assisted living, but no nursing or other care is provided. Often these are cottages on large campuses or a separate wing of the facility.

A multilevel retirement facility that has independent living units, assisted living units, and all levels of traditional nursing home care demonstrates a concept called **aging in place**. This combination of services allows the client and spouse to begin in the independent living unit. Then, if either has a need for more assistance in either the ADLs or needs nursing, the services are delivered at the same facility, so there is no need to change facilities as the need for assistance with ADL increases or health status diminishes. The multilevel facilities also have home health and hospice services.

Financing of nursing home care is primarily by Medicaid and private individuals and families. Other sources are the DVA and private insurance. Medicare only pays for skilled nursing and accounts for 10 percent of the total spent on nursing homes. Nursing homes at the intermediate level, where the largest proportion of clients is in ICF, costs $80,000 a year, depending on the level of service and location. This cost is not usually covered by any government program; it is an out-of-pocket expense borne by individuals and families.

assisted living facilities (ALFs) or Residential Care Communities Homes or apartment-like living spaces that allow for independent activities such as cooking and bathing and also provide care such as medication or treatment delivery; a nonmedical model of chronic care living arrangements.

aging in place A philosophy that allows the aging person or couple to stay in their living situation while growing older with increasing levels of personal and medical assistance as needed. These are adult living communities where the range is from individual homes to a skilled nursing facility in one complex.

How Do We Pay for LTC Services?

As you have learned in this chapter, LTC services are provided to many groups by many providers in many settings. As a consequence, it is very difficult to put a single dollar figure on the cost of LTC. As with other types of health care, payments are made by a combination of government programs such as Medicare and Medicaid and by private funding such as personal insurance and out-of-pocket payments. A great deal of LTC is unpaid assistance by family and friends.

Government Programs

The primary insurance program for the elderly, Medicare, does not pay for LTC except under narrow circumstances. If a Medicare-eligible person who has been hospitalized moves to a nursing home, Medicare will pay for the first 20 days. Between 20 and 100 days, the patient must make a daily copayment. After 100 days, no further Medicare coverage is available. Medicare also will not pay for unskilled care or long-term home care.

Medicaid will pay for nursing homes; however, the patient must meet Medicaid's income tests. The elderly often must spend down assets to become eligible, and they must do so within a time frame and in a manner that complies with Medicaid rules.

Private Funding

A great deal of information and advice is aimed at helping older Americans fund retirement, including their need for LTC services. Financial devices such as reverse mortgages and legal instruments such as living trusts are designed to protect assets in order to fund long-term living expenses. This is an area where an individual needs good professional assistance because the law changes frequently, and an uninformed decision can have devastating financial consequences (Matthews 2012).

Even those with overall good health insurance policies may not be adequately protected for a health problem that requires LTC. For this reason, LTC insurance policies have been developed. Before buying this type of policy, an individual should carefully examine it for the extent of coverage, the coverage conditions, and the exclusions. The cost of premiums should be weighed against the benefit amounts.

Some employers offer long-term disability insurance as part of their benefits package. This is insurance that will replace your income if you become disabled; it is not insurance that will pay for long-term health care.

Ethical and Political Issues in LTC

As you have seen in this chapter and previous chapters, a great number of agencies are involved in LTC. But most people are like Marge in the chapter profile and have only Medicare and Social Security benefits from the government. The person who needs more has to struggle with a very disjointed system of multiple government agencies and countless private organizations. One of the great political and health care delivery questions of the next decades is going to be how to make this system manageable and efficient and at the same time give people the assistance they need to maximize their physical/social potential and retain human dignity.

A major policy debate will be the extent to which the government should finance, regulate, and deliver LTC services. The issues here revolve around resource allocation, including the competition for funding among age groups, guardianship and medical power of attorney issues, and end-of-life care.

Resource Allocation

The ethical dilemma of who will receive society's benefits will shape much of the LTC policy debate. LTC is very resource intensive, not just monetarily but also in terms of health care professionals' efforts. Staffing ratios in LTC facilities are relatively low, especially in comparison to a general hospital, where the ratio can be over 100 people to each patient. Currently acute care is the major area funded by Medicare; as the need increases, will more resources be allocated to LTC?

If older citizens will need more resources, how do we take care of the children? Currently more children live in poverty than the 65+ age group, yet a much smaller proportion of federal spending goes to children. The elderly have powerful lobbying interests and are very politically active. After all, they can vote their interests. Children, however, have fewer spokespeople, and as a rule, they do not have the lobbying or voting clout. This makes the question of intergenerational equity very one sided.

At the family level, caregivers often face the same dilemma as policy makers. Many families are caring for both children and grandparents. For adult children, this is called the **sandwich generation**, in between the two generations.

sandwich generation The generation that is currently working and taking care of children and parents, thus sandwiched between two dependent age groups.

Health Care Power of Attorney/Guardianship

Many of the frail elderly cannot manage IADLs such as banking and health care decisions. In this case, a family member might apply to have either **medical power of attorney** for health care decisions or a full guardianship. In the health care power of attorney, the appointed family member or friend makes all the health care decisions for the elderly person. This includes treatment of acute and chronic conditions, going to an LTC facility, and end-of-life decisions.

It is easy to see that there could be some conflict between what health care providers and the decision maker would want to do. Economics could play a role in how much the family is willing to **spend down**, that is, how much money the elderly person has in assets such as a home that is available to spend for care. Should the family spend to care for the individual or should assets be conserved for the estate? This is an ethical dilemma for many families. The amount of money that families in the low- to middle-income ranges inherit has been decreasing over the last decades, in part related to spending down of assets to provide LTC.

medical power of attorney A person appointed by another who can give consent for medical care or can withhold medical care. It is a legal document that empowers the surrogate decision maker in all health care decisions if the patient is unable to make decisions.

spend down Redistributing assets so that the individual will be Medicaid eligible.

End-of-Life Decisions

Utilization statistics consistently tell us that a person uses the most care in the last 6 months of life. This statistic refers not only to the financial costs but also to the use of specialized hospitals, skilled nursing, or medical technology. The use of physician directives and living wills, along with the health care power of attorney, has become common. These tools allow the person to determine prior to an end-of-life decision what his or her wishes are concerning the use of medical technology such as ventilators, assistive cardiovascular devices such as a pacemaker, or feeding tubes.

The idea of death with dignity has a legal force at this time in several states; only Oregon has an actual assisted suicide law. These new options ideally allow the family to make very difficult decisions early in the disease process. They also give direction to caregivers. There are, of course, pros and cons concerning end-of-life decisions. There are opportunities for abuse and neglect that must be taken seriously by health care professionals. But according to many surveys, the American people want more personal control over the end-of-life process and how much technology is appropriate for the individual.

The ethical questions in LTC are complex and linked to our view of health care in general. How we treat the person who is chronically ill is a measure of our values as a country.

Career Profile: Careers in Gerontology

As you've already seen in this chapter, the older American group is the fastest-growing segment of both the general population and the health care industry. This translates into a wide variety of career options.

Gerontology is the general field of studying aging; gerontologists are specialists in the aging process across many disciplines, such as health care, sociology, psychology, and many others. So if working with this demographic appeals to you, most colleges have several departments, degrees, and certificates in age-related fields. In earlier chapters you've read about careers in clinical and non-clinical health professions, as well as various business careers related to the facilities where care is provided. There is a major shortage of people with postgraduate degrees in all fields of aging. It is a field with incredible opportunity for students at all levels.

One area you might not have considered is travel for seniors—an interesting and rapidly expanding opportunity. Recently, I went to Dominica in the Caribbean to experience firsthand this new industry. Wellness has become a magic word in the travel world. This particular program promised yoga, energy work and meditation daily, wellness-focused visits with island nutritionists, a visit with lunch to an organic farmer, hiking to pristine rain forest waterfalls, and healthy food. It was a week of interesting hikes, local food, and as promised, yoga and energy work, hikes, and water sports. All the participants were over 60.

Many spas and yoga studios are sponsoring such wellness experiences for this age group. This is an interesting development that will have several job-related spin-offs. First, the travel specialists and tour operators use people with knowledge of gerontology to help plan and market to this group.

The actual operators need some knowledge of the needs and expectations of the 60+ travelers. Travel advertising is trying to appeal to the over-60 demographic. Cruise companies like Viking show seniors experiencing the sights, enjoying cuisines, and learning new skills to entice them to join the fun. On board the program directors and tour operators cater to the needs of the client by age and mobility appropriate activities, on-board health professionals, special diets, exercise programs, and wellness activities.

Here's a few more possibilities for your exploration:

- Academia
  - Teachers and researchers at all levels
- Administration
  - Health care facilities and programs
  - Area agencies on aging
  - Government agencies
  - Human resources
  - Volunteer management—a very fast-growing field
- Financial and Legal
  - Elder law, including real estate
  - Conservators
  - Fraud prevention
  - Financial planning
  - Intergenerational issues counselors
  - Lobbyist
  - Grant writer
  - Mediator
  - Ombudsman
- Fitness and Wellness
  - Art instructor
  - Fitness trainer
  - Nutrition specialist
  - Wellness coach
  - Swimming and hydrotherapy coach
- Housing and Urban Design
  - Aging in place consultant
  - Interior designer
  - Home safety consultant
  - Real estate agent
  - Community planning specialist
  - Communal living specialist
  - Urban planner
- Leisure, Recreation, and Personal Enrichment
  - Events planner
  - Historian or genealogist
  - Athletic coaching
  - Personal services coordinator
    - Personal shopper, fashion coordinator, hair stylist, transportation facilitator, house and garden maintenance

- City, State, National, and Global Organizations
  - Specialists in aging are hired at all levels of government
  - AARP—a huge employer of people with expertise in all aspects of aging
- Private-Sector Corporations
  - Pension management
  - Health and wellness program and insurance management

Summary

The continuum of long-term care (LTC) is the network of services available to the person needing it. It may include family and friends or paid caregivers. LTC is used by anyone young or old who needs medical care or assistance with ADLs or IADLs for more than 90 days. The older American uses the majority of LTC, which is provided in the home, community-based day care centers, hospitals, assisted living centers, veterans centers, specialized hospitals, and the many levels of nursing home care. Family and friends provide about 80 percent of all LTC. The role of the government is to fund some aspects of LTC, regulate LTC providers, and provide a policy framework to ensure that the needs of this population are met.

LTC is primarily financed by individuals, either as direct payment to providers or through LTC third-party insurance. Numerous government agencies help fund LTC. The ethical and political issues in LTC revolve around the allocation of private and government resources.

Questions for Review

1. Who receives LTC in the United States?
2. To what extent are family, friends, and members of the community involved in LTC?
3. What is the relationship between IADLs and ADLs and the need for LTC?
4. Who besides the older American uses LTC, and why?
5. What are the ethical issues involved in LTC?

Questions for Discussion

1. How would you advise your congressional representative to vote on a bill to provide some level of LTC to all who need it?
2. Would you be willing to raise your taxes to pay for the care of your parents, grandparents, or a chronically ill child?
3. What LTC options are available in your community?

4. In your community, is a facility like Eola (as described in the chapter profile) available? What features are offered? What is the cost of such care? How does this cost compare to other options in your community, such as:
   a. Skilled care facility
   b. Intermediate care—regular nursing home
   c. Assisted living
   d. Foster care
   e. Specialized care such as dementia
   f. In-home care
5. Review a policy for LTC insurance. What services are covered? What is the cost?
6. Review your state's provision for a medical power of attorney. What is included?
7. What features in a continuing care community would you want for yourself and/or your family members?

Chapter References

AARP. 2009. *Caregiving in the US 2009*. Available at www.aarp.org/relationships/caregiving/info-12-2009/caregiving_ 09.html.

AARP Public Policy Institute. September 2012. *Insight on the issues.* 69.

Administration on Aging: http://www.aoa.gov.

Administration on Aging. 2014. *A profile of older Americans*. Available at http://www.aoa.acl.gov/Aging_Statistics/Profile/2014/docs/2014-Profile.pdf.

Genworth. 2015. *Cost of care overview*. Available at www.genworth.com.

Harris-Kojetin L., M. Sengupta, E. Park-Lee, and R. Valverde. 2013. *Long-term care services in the United States: 2013 overview*. National Health Care Statistics Reports; no 1. Hyattsville, MD: National Center for Health Statistics. Available at http://www.cdc.gov/nchs/data/nsltcp/long_term_care_services_2013.pdf.

Matthews, J. 2012. *Long-term care: How to plan and pay for it.* 9th ed. Berkeley, CA: NoLo Press.

United States Department of Veterans Affairs. (http://www.va.gov/budget/docs/report/2014-VAparPartII.pdf).

_____. (http://www1.va.gov/health).

For Additional Information

Administration on Aging (http://www.aoa.gov/)

American Association of Retired Persons (AARP) (www.aarp.org)

American College of Health Care Administrators (www.achca.org)

American Geriatrics Society (AGS) (www.americangeriatrics.org)

American Geriatrics Society (AGS) Foundation for Health in Aging (www.healthinaging.org)

American Society on Aging (www.asaging.org)

National Association of Area Agencies on Aging (www.n4a.org)

National Council on the Aging (www.ncoa.org)

National Hispanic Council on Aging (www.nhcoa.org)

National Institute on Aging (www.nia.nih.gov)

Older Women's League (www.owl-national.org)

9

Mental Health Services

A Combination of Systems

Learning Objectives

After reading this chapter, you should be able to:

1. Define the scope of mental illness in the United States.
2. Compare the financing of the mental health system with the general health care system.
3. Identify the major human resource sectors of the mental health system.
4. Discuss the four eras of mental health in the United States.
5. Describe the major categories of mental illness and the populations affected.
6. Discuss the ethical issues in mental health service delivery.

A Young Adult with Mental Illness

Tad is returning to college after a 5-year break because of mental illness. When he was 18 years old, he began to experience audio hallucinations. Voices in his head started to drown out the people around him. He did not tell anyone what was happening to him for two reasons: first, he was pleased to be specially chosen to hear these instructions, and second, more important, no one asked him about them.

Although he had previously led an active social life and had played in a band as a teenager, Tad became increasingly withdrawn. His parents at first thought this change in behavior was just "those teenage years." But by the time he was 19 and had dropped out of college, they were worried. At his parents' insistence, Tad saw his primary care physician. His doctor took a detailed history that included Tad's self-reported use of recreational drugs and alcohol. The doctor attributed Tad's problems to his drug and alcohol history. In the next year, however, the symptoms became worse. Tad had frequent run-ins with the police; he was homeless, unemployed, and withdrawn. Finally, Tad was arrested and jailed for vagrancy and assault.

The court asked for a psychiatric exam because of his erratic behavior in jail. Tad was diagnosed with schizophrenia and released to an emergency treatment center where he was started on psychotropic drugs. After his discharge from the center, Tad was treated on an outpatient basis. His insurance plan covered his medication and provided follow-up care through the county mental health department.

Although Tad has returned to partial functioning, he faces a lifetime of chronic illness that will need treatment. Even so, he is lucky. Because the resources of most states are stretched thin, states are often unable to provide treatment for people like Tad. The less fortunate are thus often found in homeless shelters or living on the streets.

biochemical
Involving chemical substances present in living organisms, such as dopamine.

residential care
A living arrangement in which the person resides or lives full-time at a facility.

somatic Affecting the body separate from the mind. For example, warm baths are a somatic treatment for calming the body.

talk therapy Psychotherapy invented by Sigmund Freud that involves primarily talking rather than somatic or drug therapy.

Introduction

In the United States, the mental health system evolved as a system distinct from the general medical model of health care delivery. One of the reasons it became a separate system was the stigma attached to mental illness, which caused the care to be primarily in the home and in institutions and out of the public eye until the 19th century. Other reasons include the fact that mental illness was not regarded as a physical illness (such as appendicitis) until the late 20th century, when scientists began to find a **biochemical** basis for some of the major categories of illness such as depression and schizophrenia. The treatment of mental illness at that point changed from **residential care** and physical, or **somatic**, treatments to treatments relying on drug and outpatient **talk therapy**.

This development had a profound impact on the delivery of mental health services; general practitioners and outpatient clinics could now manage mental illness. The care of people with mental illness now moved from the institutional model to a general delivery and business model like the rest of health care. In this chapter, the scope or **burden of disease**, history, diagnostic categories, delivery models, and the people who provide the services are described.

What Is Mental Illness and Mental Health?

According to the surgeon general of the United States, the term *mental illness* refers collectively to all diagnosable mental disorders. Mental disorders are health conditions characterized by alterations in thinking, **mood**, or behavior, or a combination of these associated with distress and/or impaired functioning. The precise cause, or **etiology**, of most mental disorders is not known. Researchers have found that the interactions among biological, psychological, and sociocultural factors are the major forces acting in both mental illness and mental health.

Mental health is not easily defined; like any definition of wellness, it has to be thought of in a framework that includes individual values and cultural differences. There are, however, indicators of mental health that can be assessed in an individual, such as the ability to cope with change, a positive outlook on life, the ability to interact with those close to us in a loving and supportive manner, and the general feeling of well-being. The mental health system addresses both mental health and illness with a wide variety of professionals, government and private programs, and **delivery models**.

Examples of mental illness include **mood disorders**, such as **major depression; cognitive**, or thinking, disorders, such as **Alzheimer's disease**; and behavior disorders, such as **eating disorders**. Mental illness is clinically diagnosed using a system that takes into consideration the observable signs and symptoms of the illness, the course and duration of the illness, the response to treatment, and the functional impairment caused by the illness. In the United States, mental illness is diagnosed by using the American Psychiatric Association's *Diagnostic and Statistical Manual of Mental Disorders*. It was first published in 1952; the current version is DSM-V-TR-2013. This manual is updated every several years and establishes the criteria for a mental illness diagnosis. The manual is rapidly becoming the major diagnostic tool for mental illness around the globe.

These criteria are difficult to measure in absolutely objective terms, so the tracking of mental illness is not an exact science. The two best-known comprehensive studies attempting to track the behavior and feelings of mentally ill people are the *National Comorbidity Survey* and the *Epidemiological Catchment Area* study. Both studies relied on extensive interviews to establish mental illness patterns.

Scope of Mental Illness

Mental illness is a global problem. It impacts the daily lives of the afflicted individuals and their family, friends, and employers, as well as the community as a whole. The World Health Organization (WHO) estimates that 400 million people suffer globally from depression. That is a population close to the total number of Americans. Further an estimated 60 million suffer from bipolar disease, 21 million from schizophrenia, and 35 million from dementia

burden of disease The cost of a disease in terms of the individual, family, and community disability, including lost work, family relationships, and community participation.

mood The state of mind experienced at a particular time.

etiology The study of the causes and origins of disease.

mental health The ability to cope with change, a positive outlook on life, ability to interact in close relationships in a loving and supportive manner, and the general feeling of well-being that can be assessed in the individual.

delivery models Systems to bring a type of care to individuals and groups.

mood disorders An altered state of mind, such as the continuous sadness known as depression.

major depression A depression that lasts for a significant period of time or recurs frequently; a medical diagnosis.

cognitive Relating to the process of thinking or acquiring knowledge. Cognitive diseases disrupt the ability to acquire or remember knowledge.

Alzheimer's disease
A degenerative disorder that affects the brain and causes dementia.

eating disorders
A group of diseases that describes a patient's focus on food, obsessive eating, or not eating, along with faulty perception of body image.

(http://www.who.int/healthinfo/statistics/en/). The WHO estimates that 70–80 percent of people afflicted with a mental disorder receive no treatment.

The availability and quality of mental health services affect every family and employer in the United States. Most mental illness is a chronic lifetime disease that interferes with an individual's ability to participate fully in family life, work, and school. Mental illness strikes one out of every five adults, or about 26 percent of the population. This figure includes both mental illness diagnosis and substance abuse. Approximately 19 percent of the adult population has a diagnosis of mental illness. Substance abuse of drugs and/or alcohol occurs in about 6 percent of the adult population. Dual diagnoses of both mental illness and substance abuse are responsible for the final 3 percent. This translates to 57.7 million adults in any given year. Mental disorders are the leading cause of disability in both the United States and Canada for ages 15 to 44.

For children, the figures are not as well documented, but it is estimated that mild mental functional impairment occurs in 20 percent of children. Serious emotional disturbance is found in 9 percent of children between ages 9 and 17.

Serious psychological distress (SPD) is a category that includes mental health problems severe enough to cause moderate to serious impairment in social, occupational, or school functioning and to require treatment. This is tracked by the National Health Interview Survey (NHIS). In 2013 this survey found that women were more likely to have SPD than men, uninsured more likely than insured; as income increased SPD decreased, and one-quarter of those over 65 so afflicted had limitations in activities of daily living (ADLs). Further it demonstrated that those with SPD were more likely to have chronic obstructive pulmonary disease, heart disease, and diabetes (http://www.cdc.gov/nchs/data/databriefs/db203.pdf).

It is further estimated that only about half the people who have mental illness get adequate treatment. Part of this is because of economic and insurance status, cultural barriers, and the stigma of mental illness, and part is related to the inadequacy of the system itself. However, the implementation of the Affordable Care Act together with the Mental Health Parity and Addiction Equity Act has already afforded an additional 60 million Americans mental health services (SAMHSA's CFRI Financing Focus - financing-focus-06152015.pdf).

Financing the System

The total cost for the mental health system accounts for about 6 percent of all the dollars spent on health care, which translates to over $115 billion in the United States. The system is funded by a combination of public spending, third-party insurance, and individual out-of-pocket spending. Among the public payers, the bulk of the funds comes from Medicaid, followed by other state and local agencies, Medicare, and other federal programs such as those offered through the Department of Veterans Affairs. The total world expenditure on mental health is expected to top $6 trillion by 2030. These figures do not include lost time and earnings opportunities, which are estimated at 35 percent of GDP worldwide (http://www.samhsa.gov/sites/default/files/samhsa-fy2016-congressional-justification.pdf).

During the past two decades, there have been important shifts in which parties are responsible for mental health funding. Direct state funding of mental health care has been reduced, whereas Medicaid funding of mental health care has grown in relative importance. In part this is because of the substantial funding available to the states through the Medicaid program and public health block grants by the federal government. One consequence of this shift is that the Medicaid program design influences the delivery of each state's mental health care. In addition, the Mental Health Parity and Addiction Equity Act and the Affordable Care Act have significantly increased the number of people who have access to mental health care. This legislation is also impacting delivery methods. Traditional state mental health agencies and departments of health and human services, however, continue to be an important force in making public mental health services policy.

Mental disorders and substance abuse are linked for diagnostic and cost accounting purposes, but both third-party payers and providers handle them differently. A majority of private health insurance plans have a benefit that combines coverage of mental illness and substance abuse. However, many of the treatment services for mental illness and for substance abuse are separate and use different types of providers. The same is true for virtually all the public funds for these services. This separation causes problems for treating the substantial proportion of individuals with both mental illness and substance abuse disorders who would otherwise benefit if both disorders were treated together.

Private insurance coverage has played a somewhat more limited role in mental health financing in the past decade. Various cost containment efforts have been pursued in the private sector through the introduction of managed care. This trend has increased the use of the general medical/primary care sector for mental health care. At the same time, private insurance coverage for prescription drugs has expanded dramatically. As a result of these efforts, insurance coverage for mental health drug therapy is moving toward parity with coverage for other illnesses.

The parity of payment to consumers is a major goal of mental health legislation. The Mental Health Parity and Addiction Equity Act and the Affordable Health Care Act both target this concept. **Parity** refers to the effort to treat mental health financing on the same basis or on par with financing for general health services. The fundamental motivation behind parity legislation is the desire to cover mental illness like any other physical disease. A parity mandate requires all insurers in a market to offer the same coverage, but as of 2006 only a handful of states required parity.

parity Equality; in this context it means equality of benefits between insurance coverage for mental health and medical coverage.

Organizing the Mental Health System

The U.S. mental health system is not a unified system at all. In this chapter, the *mental health system* means all services to those with a mental illness diagnosis, substance abuse, dementia, and children who have either cognitive impairment or a mental illness diagnosis. There are four ways to categorize this so-called system: (1) by who delivers services, (2) by treatment types, (3) by care setting, and (4) by human resource components.

Who Delivers Services

Mental health services can be provided by a wide variety of individuals from non-clinical self-help volunteers to psychiatrists. State and federal regulations vary widely on who can deliver services to people with mental health issues. Insurance companies reimburse some types of therapists and not others.

Treatment Types

Another way to categorize the system is by treatment types. These can include self-help, psychotherapy, talk therapy, behavioral therapy, drug therapy, and somatic device therapy such as electroshock therapy.

Care Settings

The mental health system is also defined by care settings. These include home care, community-based residential care, day care, sheltered work settings, outpatient facilities, and private psychiatric and recovery institutions. Care settings can even include public institutions for emergency and long-term care.

Human Resource Components

A common way to categorize the system is by its four major human resources components: the specialty mental health sector, the general medical/primary care sector, the human services sector, and the voluntary support network. This method of categorizing is popular because it recognizes that mental health problems are treated by a large variety of people who work in many different settings. The surgeon general's report on mental health estimates that these mental health sectors serve about 11 percent of the overall health care services provided in a year.

The specialty mental health sector includes mental health professionals such as psychiatrists, psychologists, counselors, psychiatric nurses, and psychiatric social workers. These professionals practice primarily in specialized mental health clinics, public and private psychiatric hospitals, and psychiatric beds in general hospitals. They also coordinate a wide variety of services to the seriously mentally ill through case management. It is estimated that 6 percent of adults and 8 percent of children access mental health care through this sector.

The general medical/primary care sector is composed of health care professionals such as primary care physicians, general internists, and nurse practitioners who practice in offices, general hospitals, and long-term care facilities. They are often the first health care provider contacted by an adult suffering from mental illness. Because the use of psychoactive drugs by primary care professionals has become widespread, adults with mild to moderate disease may use only this sector. Fewer children than adults use these professionals: only 3 percent as compared to 6 percent of adults.

The major sector that assesses, diagnoses, and treats childhood mental illness and cognitive disorders is the human services sector. Social services, school-based counseling, residential rehabilitation services, vocational rehabilitation, criminal justice/prison-based services, and religious counselors all belong to this sector. The school-based services are used by 16 percent of children, and child welfare and juvenile justice systems serve another 3 percent.

The last of the four sectors is the voluntary support network sector. Self-help groups, such as Alcoholics Anonymous (AA) and Al-Anon, and peer counseling are a rapidly growing part of the mental health services sector. There are 12-step type programs for many diagnoses, including those in the substance abuse category.

History of Mental Health Care in the United States

The history of mental health care demonstrates a shift in perception. Historically mental illness was seen as a problem of possession by evil spirits or as an imbalance in vital elements. Melancholy, now known as depression, was considered an imbalance in the vital humors until modern times. Epilepsy was a sign that visions and spirits visited the person. Freud began the modern era of psychiatry with what we now call psychotherapy or talk therapy. More important, he began to characterize the symptoms of mental illness. We still use a variant of the system Freud began over 100 years ago.

As the perception shifted from illness to wellness, so did the delivery systems for care. Prior to the 1950s, the emphasis was on housing people who were the most seriously mentally ill. The institutions for them were at best the sanatorium model where patients were housed comfortably but not allowed to leave. Some of these were very luxurious. At the other end of the spectrum were the huge charity and state-run institutions where people with mental illness were literally thrown into huge cells and food was pushed through doors. No attempt was made to cure or to see the individual as anything but subhuman.

The history of mental health care in the United States can be divided into four eras, each focused on reforming the problems not previously addressed. The four are the moral treatment era, the mental hygiene era, the community mental health era, and the current community support era (see Table 9.1).

Table 9.1	*Historical Reform Movements in Mental Health Treatment in the United States*

Reform Movement	Era	Setting	Focus of Reform
Moral treatment	1800–1850	Asylum	Humane restorative treatment
Mental hygiene	1890–1920	Mental hospital or clinic	Prevention, scientific orientation
Community mental health	1955–1970	Community mental health centers	Deinstitutionalization, social integration
Community support	1975–present	Community support	Mental illness as a social welfare problem (e.g., housing, employment)

Source: U.S. Department of Health and Human Services. 1999. *Mental health: A report of the surgeon general.* Rockville, MD: U.S. Department of Health and Human Services, Substance Abuse and Mental Health Services Administration, Center for Mental Health Services, National Institutes of Health, National Institute of Mental Health, Table 2.9.

The Moral Era

An era of "moral treatment" was introduced from Europe at the turn of the 19th century, representing the first of four reform movements in mental health services in the United States.

The first reformers, including Dorothea Dix and Horace Mann, imported the idea from Europe that mental illness could be treated by removing the individual to an asylum to receive a mix of somatic (physical treatment like baths, exercise, and special diet) and psychosocial treatments in a controlled environment characterized by "moral" sensibilities. The term *moral* had a different connotation than that of today. Then it meant the return of the individual to reason by the application of psychologically oriented therapy.

The building of private and public asylums characterized the moral treatment period. Almost every state had an asylum dedicated to the early treatment of mental illness to restore mental health and to keep patients from becoming chronically ill. Moral treatment accomplished the former objective, but it could not prevent chronic illness.

Mental Hygiene Era

Shortly after the Civil War, the failure of the early treatment moral era was recognized. Asylums were built for the untreatable chronic patients. The quality of care deteriorated in public institutions, where overcrowding and underfunding were the norm. A new reform movement, devoted to mental hygiene, as it was called, began in the late 19th century. It combined the newly emerging concepts of public health (which at the time was referred to as "hygiene"), scientific medicine, and social progressivism. Although the states built the public asylums, local governments were expected to pay for each episode of care. To avoid the expense, many communities continued to use local almshouses and jails for the mentally ill person. Asylums could not maintain their budgets, care deteriorated, and newspaper exposés revealed inhuman conditions both in asylums and in local welfare institutions.

The care of individuals with mental illness became the responsibility of state governments with the passage of the State Care Acts, passed between 1894 and World War I. Local government took the opportunity to send everyone with a mental illness, including dependent older citizens, to state asylums. Dementia was redefined as a mental illness, although only some of the older residents were demented. For the past century, the states carried this responsibility at very low cost, despite the magnitude of the task. This was accomplished by centralizing the care into one or two state mental hospitals that cared for thousands of residents at a time. The movie *One Flew over the Cuckoo's Nest* depicts life in such a hospital.

The reformers of the mental hygiene period formed the National Committee on Mental Hygiene (now the National Mental Health Association, NMHA) and called for an expansion of the new science, particularly neuropathology, in asylums, which were renamed mental hospitals. They also called for "psychopathic hospitals and clinics" to bring the new science to patients in smaller institutions associated with medical schools. They opened several psychiatric units in general hospitals to move mental health care into the mainstream of health care. The mental hygienists believed in the principles of early treatment and expected to prevent chronic mental illness. To support this effort, they advocated for outpatient treatment to identify early cases of mental disorder and to follow discharged patients.

Early treatment was no more successful in preventing patients from becoming chronically ill in the early 20th century than it was in the early years of the previous century. At best, the hospitals provided humane custodial care; at worst, they neglected or abused the patients. Length of stay did begin to decline for newly admitted patients, but older long-stay patients filled public asylums. Financial problems and overcrowding deepened during the Depression and during World War II.

Community Mental Health Movement

Enthusiasm for early interventions, developed by military mental health services during World War II, brought a new sense of optimism about treatment by the middle of the 20th century. Again, early treatment of mental disorders was championed; a new concept, community mental health, was born. The NMHA figured prominently in this reform, along with the Group for the Advancement of Psychiatry. Borrowing some ideas from the mental hygienists and capitalizing on the advent of new drugs for treating psychosis and depression, community mental health reformers argued that they could bring mental health services to the public in their communities. They suggested that long-term institutional care in mental hospitals had been neglectful, ineffective, and even harmful. The joint policies of community care and deinstitutionalization led to dramatic declines in the length of hospital stay and the discharge of many patients from custodial care in hospitals (U.S. Department of Health and Human Services 1999).

The Current Mental Health System: The Community Support Movement

The past 25 years have been marked by discrete defining trends in the mental health field, according to the Surgeon General's *Report on Mental Health*. There has been an extraordinary increase in the pace and productivity of scientific research on the brain and behavior. The introduction of a range of effective treatments for most mental disorders has changed clinical and client response dramatically.

In the modern era, the care of mentally ill people is decentralized. No longer do we have huge institutions that served as permanent homes for those diagnosed with mental illness and neurological disorders. The mental institutions of the 1950s and 1960s housed thousands of patients; those same institutions today house only a few hundred patients with the most serious mental illnesses. The number of people with mental illness in the community has not changed to any great degree, but the treatment is now outpatient and in small group homes.

With the deinstitutionalization of people committed to psychiatric hospitals and changes in psychiatric treatment brought about by psychoactive drugs and managed care efforts, consumers developed self-help programs designed to improve outcomes for people with mental illness through peer support. Services offered include drop-in centers, vocational and housing programs, peer counseling, case-management services, crisis alternatives to hospitalizations, advocacy training, business ventures, and peer support groups. Although these programs have existed for over two decades, little formal evaluation has focused on the effectiveness of this mental health delivery model. A better understanding of existing consumer-operated service programs is needed to provide the empirical basis for creating effective partnerships between these programs and traditional services.

Major Categories of Mental Illness

The scope and distribution of the most frequently occurring mental illness diagnoses are described here to provide a concrete idea of the wide variety of illnesses the mental health system addresses. According to the National Institute of Mental Health, the major categories of mental illness are mood disorders, schizophrenia, obsessive-compulsive disorders, anxiety disorders, posttraumatic stress disorder (PTSD), suicide, and cognitive impairments. Major depression is the leading cause of disability worldwide for people older than 5 years. For women, the major causes of disability are depression, schizophrenia, and bipolar disease. Many people suffer from dual disorder (more than one mental illness diagnosis). Table 9.2, "Major Mental Illness Categories at a Glance," will give you information about the types of mental illness, who is affected, and treatments.

Table 9.2	*Major Mental Illness Categories at a Glance*				
Disorder	**Description/ Symptoms**	**Demographics**	**Age of Onset**	**Treatment**	**Notes**
Mood disorders, Major Depressive Disorder, Dysthymic Disorder, Bipolar Disorder	Prolonged sadness, changes in sleep and appetite, irritability, feelings of guilt and anxiety	Affects 9.5% of adult Americans— 20.9 million, affects twice as many women as men, often co-occur with anxiety disorders and substance abuse	Between 15 and 30, median age 25–32, diagnosis in very young children and older people more common in last decade	Cognitive behavioral therapy, psychotherapy, social supportive care, pharma-cotherapy: antiepressants, tranquilizers, mood stabilizers, sleep aids, or sedative mediation	Same genes suspected in both depression and bipolar disease
Suicide	90% have a diagnosable depressive disorder or substance abuse	In 2006, 33,300 people died, highest rates in white men over age 85, four times as many men as women	From early adolescence to old age	**PREVENTION** ***Any person who talks about killing him/herself needs help. If you or anyone you know is considering suicide get help! Life Line – 1800273 8255 is avail-able 24/7 to anyone free***	Women attempt suicide three times more often than men. It is estimated that there are as many as 25 suicide attempts for every death
Schizophrenia	Loss of contact with reality, severe disturbance in social functioning, bizarre thoughts, withdrawal from social interactions, hallucinations, delusions	2.4 million adults age 18 and older, affects men and women with equal frequency, if one twin exhibits symptoms the other has a 45% chance of at some time becoming symptomatic	Men—appears in late teens or early twenties. Women—in twenties or early thirties. Over 10,000 new cases are diagnosed every year	Pharmaco-therapy: antipsychotic primarily, anti-depressants, psychosocial treatments	Genes are being identi-fied, but no specific set has been found. It seems that both a genetic predisposition and an environ-mental stressor are needed to trigger symptoms

(continued)

Table 9.2	*Major Mental Illness Categories at a Glance (continued)*				
Disorder	Description/ Symptoms	Demographics	Age of Onset	Treatment	Notes
Anxiety	Heightened feelings of dread, fear, apprehension, worry and/or uneasiness	13% of adults between 18 and 54 suffer an anxiety disorder		Psychotherapy and cognitive behavioral therapy; pharmaco-therapy, tranquilizers, and sleep aids	Common to have more than one anxiety disorder coupled with substance abuse
Anxiety—Panic	Sudden onset of intense anx-iety coupled with physical symptoms like hyperven-tilating and tachycardia	2.4 million Americans 18–54	Late adolescence or early adulthood	As above plus treatment for physical symptoms	About one in three people with panic attacks develop agoraphobia—afraid of open spaces
Anxiety— Obsessive-Compulsive	Anxiety disorder characterized by recurrent, unwanted thoughts (obsessions) and/or repetitive behavior (compulsions)	2.2 million Americans age 18 and older	Symptoms may begin in early childhood or adolescence, median age of onset is 19	Pharmacother-apy, exposure psychotherapy, social support groups, and deep brain stimulation	
Anxiety— Posttraumatic stress	Develops after a terrifying ordeal that involved physical harm or the threat of harm. Flashbacks of the incident occur frequently, causing intense stress	Affects about 7.7 million Americans. Affect women more than men. Some evidence of family susceptibility	Any age after a traumatic event	Pharmacother-apy, psycho-therapy, and social support groups all are effective	It often manifests with-in 3 months of the event, but may not surface for years. Often accompanied by depression, substance abuse, and other anxieties

Table 9.2	*(continued)*				
Disorder	**Description/ Symptoms**	**Demographics**	**Age of Onset**	**Treatment**	**Notes**
Eating— Anorexia nervosa, bulimia, binge eating	Anorexia— Fear of obesity and ritualistic food practices, loss of 15% of body weight, excessive dieting and self-induced vomiting. Bulimia— massive binge eating, use of laxatives and vomiting	Females 15–24 0.5%–3.7% of females experience anorexia and 1%–4.2% bulimia, while 2–5% of all Americans experience binge-eating disorder	35% of cases are male; mortality among people with anorexia is 12 times higher than the annual death rate of 15–24-year-olds from all other causes combined	Emergency medical maintenance for complications. Cognitive behavioral therapy, psychotherapy, social supportive care, pharmacotherapy: antidepressants	Bulimia had the highest morbidity—the purging may permanently damage the GI system and teeth. A colostomy may be needed, and death may be caused by cardiac arrhythmias
Attention Deficit Hyperactivity (ADHD)	Inattention and/or hyperactivity and impulsivity	Most common mental disorder in children, also affects 4.1% of adults 18–44. Affects males more often than females	Becomes evident in preschool or early elementary years, median age of onset is 7 years old	Pharmacotherapy: stimulants, cognitive behavioral therapy, counseling, collaboration between providers and school/family/ friends/ employee	Etiology unknown, but twin studies suggest genetic susceptibility
Autism	Deficits in reciprocal language and social interactions, characterized by repetitive stereotyped behaviors— minimal eye contact, delayed language, disinterest in social interactions	Prevalence estimates difficult due to difference in the ways that cases are identified and defined, differences in study methods, and changes in diagnostic criteria. But 3–4 cases per 1,000 children is an acceptable estimate	Generally diagnosed by age 3. Four times more common in boys, but when girls affected symptoms are more severe and with greater cognitive impairment	No specific medications are approved for ASDs, but medications for behavior and mood may be used. Applied behavior analysis— individual intense one-to-one therapy has been shown to improve behavior and communication skills	Part of a group known as autism spectrum disorders (ASDs), autism being the most debilitating form, Asperger's syndrome produces milder symptoms

(continued)

Table 9.2	*Major Mental Illness Categories at a Glance (continued)*				
Disorder	**Description/ Symptoms**	**Demographics**	**Age of Onset**	**Treatment**	**Notes**
Alzheimer's disease	Progressive form of dementia that seriously disrupts activities of daily living, behavior, and mood	Affects 4.5 million Americans; this number has doubled since 1980. Most common cause of dementia 65 and older. Increasing age is greatest risk factor	Symptoms first appear after 65, 1 in 10 individuals over 65 and nearly half of those over 85 are affected	Medications can slow progression and treat associated symptoms of depression, anxiety, and aggression. Social supports and occupational and physical therapy are important	From time of diagnosis, people with AD survive about half as long as those of similar age without dementia. Life span after diagnosis 8–10 years. Rare inherited forms can strike as early as 30s–40s.

Source: National Institute of Mental Health. *The numbers count: Mental disorders in America*. Bethesda, MD: National Institute of Mental Health, available at www.nimh.nih.gov/health/publications/the-numbers-count-mental-disorders-in-america/index.shtml.

Risk Factors and Prevention

Risk factors are those characteristics or hazards that, if present for a given individual, make it more likely that this individual, rather than someone selected at random, will develop a disorder. Some risks such as gender and family history are fixed; that is, the individual cannot change them. Other risk factors, such as a lack of social support, inability to read, and exposure to bullying, can be altered by strategic and potent interventions. Current research is focusing on the interplay between biological risk factors and psychological risk factors and how they can be modified. As explained earlier, even with a highly heritable condition such as schizophrenia, studies have shown that in over half of identical twins, the second twin does not have schizophrenia. This suggests the possibility of modifying the environment to eventually prevent the biological risk factor (i.e., the unidentified gene that contributes to schizophrenia) from being expressed.

Because mental health is so closely related to all other aspects of health, it is important to look at all the different types of interaction among the biological, psychological, and sociocultural factors. For example, chronic illness, unemployment, substance abuse, racism, and violence can be risk factors or mediating variables for the onset of mental health problems. Yet some of the same factors can also be related to the consequences of mental health problems (e.g., depression may lead to substance abuse, which in turn may lead to lung or liver cancer).

Suicide Prevention

Any person who talks about killing him or herself needs help!!!!

    If you or anyone you know is considering suicide, get help!

Life Line—1 800 273 8255 is available 24/7 to anyone free.

Treatment

Mental disorders are treatable; new brain-based research increases the ability to diagnose and treat mental illness every day. A number of treatments are available that diminish symptoms and increase functionality. In fact, for most mental disorders, there is generally not just one but a range of treatments of proven value to patients. Most treatments fall under two general categories: psychosocial and pharmacological. Moreover, the combination of the two—known as multimodal therapy—can sometimes be even more effective than each individually.

    The evidence for treatment being more effective than placebo is overwhelming. The degree of effectiveness tends to vary depending on the disorder and the target population. What is optimal for one disorder and/or age group may not be optimal for another. Furthermore, treatments generally need to be tailored to the client and to client preferences (http://www.samhsa.gov/topics/behavioral-health-treatments-services).

    If treatment is so effective, then why are so few people receiving it? Studies reveal that less than a third of adults with a diagnosable mental disorder, and even a smaller proportion of children, receive any mental health services in a given year. Systemic barriers, economics, stigma of disease, and cultural responses all contribute to the underutilization for persons with mental illness. The single largest barrier is socioeconomic class. The working poor and the underinsured have a very difficult time accessing adequate assessment and treatment. It is only in recent decades that the government has become the primary resource for mental health services.

Ethical Issues in Mental Health

The issues surrounding confidentiality, barriers to mental health services, parity in financing mental health and general health, and the uninsured are all ethical questions as well as policy questions. The ability of an individual or family to access mental health services is critical to the quality of life for the person with a mental illness as well as his or her family and social network, which makes access a key ethical issue when talking about the delivery of mental health services.

The barriers that are culturally and ethnically centered require us to take action to decrease these barriers. This would include decreasing racism, looking at poverty as both an economic and an ethical issue, and reducing the stigma of mental illness. Only when these underlying causes have been addressed can we begin to have a system that is ethically responsive.

Another major issue in mental health services is confidentiality. Although it is also an important issue in general health care, there are special considerations in the mental health area. An individual with a mental illness might decide not to seek treatment for many reasons. Some might forgo treatment for financial reasons. Others might decide that the risk of stigma and discrimination still encountered by people with mental illness is too high a risk. Many people pay directly to the mental health provider rather than use the insurance provided by their employer because of fear that if it were known they had a mental illness, they would be fired or not considered for promotion.

Career Profile: Mental Health

Would you like to help someone like Tad? The fields of mental health and behavioral health offer many opportunities. A person can begin as mental health aide and progress to psychologist, psychiatrist, or researcher. Education requirements range from on-the-job training to doctorates. Most of the counseling and social service jobs require a minimum of a bachelor's and in most cases, a master's degree and state licensing. Salaries start in the $40,000–$50,000 range. The upward career path is in management or private practice. The mental health career field is overwhelming female, with less than 20 percent of practitioners being male.

The enactment of the Affordable Care Act has greatly expanded the demand for mental health counselors at all levels and will provide for a strong job market for years to come. In addition, the increase in the number of veterans has also stimulated demand.

The mental counselor assesses, diagnoses, and treats mental health issues in a variety of settings. Most commonly they are found in public health, the Veterans Administration, the Department of Defense, community mental health departments, rehabilitation facilities, inpatient mental health facilities, outpatient departments of hospitals, and increasingly in private practice or a group practice with other mental health specialists such as psychiatrists and psychologists.

Clinical social work, bereavement counseling, gender counseling, trauma counseling, case management, community health, and clinical psychology are other fields that provide similar services to clients.

A position listing for a licensed mental health counselor with the Department of Veterans Affairs indicates some of the job duties and requirements:

The purpose of the Readjustment Counseling Service is to assist combat veterans who have not achieved an adequate readjustment to civilian life after military service. Veterans eligible for Vet Center services include all combat/conflict veterans (Operation Iraqi Freedom/ Operation New Dawn, Operation Enduring Freedom, Vietnam era, Lebanon, Grenada, Panama conflicts, Persian Gulf, Korea, and Somalia, WWII) and families. The incumbent's primary responsibility is to provide clinical/therapeutic services and readjustment counseling to eligible veterans and their significant others. He/ she works within the guidelines provided by the Team Leader to provide effective services including, but not limited to individual, group, conjoint, vocational, educational, substance abuse and readjustment counseling. Incumbent independently conducts intake and needs assessment of eligible veterans and their significant others. The Counseling Therapist provides crisis intervention, psycho/ social counseling therapy and assists with acute psychiatric emergencies. Incumbent develops veteran's employability, provides assistance and referral regarding Agent Orange and Persian Gulf Syndrome. The Counseling Therapist is also responsible for the presentation of educational programs and actively participates in program planning and development, making recommendations in program policies and procedures.

The position requires "experience with directly engaging and providing treatment to traumatized combat veterans exhibiting complex and diversified psychosocial problems and mental health issues, including posttraumatic stress disorder, homelessness, avoidant and those exhibiting anger/ rage reactions. Experience with direct provision of clinical interventions to family/significant others of traumatized veterans, including spouses/ partners, minor and teenaged children exhibiting effects of secondary PTSD, PTSD, and other family related difficulties" (www.usajobs.gov/GetJob/ ViewDetails/405460700).

Summary

Mental illness is a significant health concern in the United States; one in five Americans has a mental disorder in any given year, and 15 percent of the adult population use some form of mental health services during the year. In addition to adults, 21 percent of children ages 9 to 17 receive mental health services in a given year. The major categories of mental illness include mood disorders, schizophrenia, obsessive-compulsive disorders, anxiety disorders, PTSD, suicide, and cognitive impairments. The history of mental health treatment has moved from warehousing to individual treatment with a sophisticated mix of drugs and psychotherapy. The current mental health service system is complex and connects many sectors. As a result, care may become organizationally fragmented, creating barriers to access. The system is also financed from many funding streams, adding to the complexity. Although the United States spends $99 billion on the direct treatment of mental disorders, substance abuse, and Alzheimer's disease, there is concern that mental illness does not receive the equivalent amount of spending that physical illnesses receive. Parity legislation attempts to resolve this issue. In addition to access and resource allocation, there are ethical issues regarding confidentiality and discrimination.

Questions for Review

1. Define mental health.
2. Describe the most common mental health conditions in children, adolescents, adults, and the elderly.
3. Compare the role of the individual patient, insurance companies, and the state and federal government in paying for mental health services.
4. Describe the current system used to deliver mental health services in the United States.
5. Compare and contrast the treatment for mental illness from the 1880s to the present.
6. Refer to the profile at the beginning of this chapter. How common is Tad's diagnosis, and whom does it most commonly affect?

Questions for Discussion

1. Why is it so difficult to define mental health?
2. Do you believe that there is still a stigma attached to mental illness? What other factors might prevent a person from seeking treatment?
3. What mental health care facilities are available at your college?
4. Should mental health and substance abuse be treated together?
5. Should insurance treat mental health treatment the same way it treats any other illnesses?
6. Refer to the profile at the beginning of this chapter. Discuss Tad's case from two perspectives: as if he were your friend and if he were a stranger you heard talking to himself on the streets. How would you react differently? What is the general feeling about people who have hallucinations or talk to themselves? Do you think this perception exists in all cultures?
7. What is society's obligation to people with mental health problems, and how has that changed over the last 200 years?

Chapter References

http://www.who.int/mediacentre/factsheets/fs396/en/
http://www.who.int/healthinfo/global_burden_disease/metrics_daly/en/
http://www.cdc.gov/nchs/fastats/mental-health.htm
http://www.cdc.gov/nchs/data/databriefs/db203.pdf
http://www.samhsa.gov/health-financing/implementation-mental-health-parity-addiction-equity-act
http://www.nimh.nih.gov/about/director/2011/the-global-cost-of-mental-illness.shtml

https://www.healthcare.gov/

http://www.samhsa.gov/data/

http://www.census.gov/quickfacts/table/AGE775213/00

http://www.samhsa.gov/health-financing

http://www.census.gov/newsroom/cspan/mental_illness/20130315_cspan_mental_illness_12.pdf

http://www.samhsa.gov/data/sites/default/files/CBHSQ-DR-C11-MI-Mortality-2014/CBHSQ-DR-C11-MI-Mortality-2014.pdf

National Institute of Mental Health. 2009. *The numbers count: Mental disorders in America*. Bethesda, MD: National Institute of Mental Health (http://www.lb7.uscourts.gov/documents/12-cv-1072url2.pdf).

Substance Abuse and Mental Health Services Administration (www.samhsa.gov).

U.S. Department of Health and Human Services. 1999. *Mental health: A report of the surgeon general*. Rockville, MD: U.S. Department of Health and Human Services, Substance Abuse and Mental Health Services Administration, Center for Mental Health Services, National Institutes of Health, National Institute of Mental Health, Table 2.9.

For Additional Information

Mental Health Disorders—statistics (www.cdc.gov/nchs/fastats/mental.htm)

National Institute of Mental Health (www.nimh.nih.gov)

National Institute of Mental Health. n.d. *Schizophrenia*. Bethesda, MD: National Institute of Mental Health (http://www.nimh.nih.gov/health/topics/schizophrenia/index.shtml).

10

The Public Health System

The Government's Role

Learning Objectives

After reading this chapter, you should be able to:

1. Define the concept of public health and give examples of public health activities.

2. Explain the role of government in public health.

3. List two or more national (federal) public health agencies.

4. Explain the role of boards of public health and licensing/regulatory boards.

5. Describe at least one major government initiative to protect the public's health.

6. Identify the key reporting obligations that health professionals are mandated to uphold.

Ebola—A National and Worldwide Public Health Crisis

The 2014 Ebola epidemic was the largest outbreak in history, affecting multiple countries in West Africa, the United States (11 cases), and Europe (15 cases). Over 27,000 cases and 11,000 deaths were reported. The World Health Organization (WHO) believes the number of deaths was underestimated due to the difficulty in tracking cases in West Africa.

Ebola, previously known as Ebola hemorrhagic fever, is a rare and deadly disease caused by infection with one of the five Ebola virus strains. Ebola can cause disease in humans and nonhuman primates (monkeys, gorillas, and chimpanzees). Ebola viruses are found in several African countries. Ebola was first discovered in 1976 near the Ebola River in the Democratic Republic of the Congo. Since then, outbreaks have appeared sporadically in Africa. The 2014 outbreak was larger and caused more deaths than all other known outbreaks combined.

People get Ebola through direct contact (through broken skin or mucous membranes in, for example, the eyes, nose, or mouth) with:

- Blood or body fluids (including, but not limited to, urine, saliva, sweat, feces, vomit, breast milk, and semen) of a person who is sick with or has died from Ebola
- Objects (like needles and syringes) that have been contaminated with body fluids from a person who is sick with Ebola or the body of a person who has died from Ebola
- Infected fruit bats or primates (apes and monkeys)
- Possibly from contact with semen from a man who has recovered from Ebola (for example, by having oral, vaginal, or anal sex)

In the United States, the Centers for Disease Control (CDC) and its partners took precautions to prevent additional Ebola cases in the United States. There were 102 teams on exclusive Ebola assignment in the United States. In addition, thousands of CDC staff members provided logistics, staffing, communication, analytics, management, and other support functions. For example, the CDC prepared U.S. health care facilities to safely manage a patient with suspected Ebola. Updated infection control guidance for health care workers was put on the CDC webpage.

Introduction

As individuals, our health is important to us. Yet even though we take care of ourselves, we don't live alone or in isolation. Society is made up of millions of individuals. What affects one member of a community can often affect another member. The health of the nation is the responsibility of the public health system in the United States.

In this chapter, you'll learn about the public health system in the United States: what it is and who's responsible. The history and basic activities of public health are discussed, and the role of government in public health is described. Finally, you'll learn about the challenges facing public health in the 21st century. The public health system is not a single system. It is made up of many different agencies coming together to improve the health and lives of Americans. This is a brief overview, highlighting some of the major components of the system.

The spread of disease by travelers was of particular concern. The CDC recommended that travelers entering the United States from Guinea, Liberia, and Sierra Leone be actively monitored by state and local health departments. Additional public health actions were recommended depending on travelers' possible exposures to Ebola while in one of the three countries. The CDC and Customs and Border Protection (CBP) conducted enhanced entry screening at five U.S. airports (New York's JFK International, Washington–Dulles, Newark, Chicago–O'Hare, and Atlanta) for all U.S.–bound air travelers who had been in Guinea, Liberia, or Sierra Leone. A Check and Report Ebola (CARE) Kit for travelers arriving in the United States from these countries was developed that included information about Ebola, tools to help travelers check their temperature and symptoms each day for 21 days, and information about who to call if they have symptoms. Ebola-specific travel messages for electronic monitors to reach travelers from West Africa and posters for TSA screening areas of airports to reach outbound travelers were developed and posted.

The CDC worked with airlines to address crew and airline staff concerns while ensuring the ability of humanitarian and public health organizations to transport assistance into countries with widespread Ebola transmission. It also worked with airlines, airports, ministries of health, and other partners in West Africa to provide technical assistance for conducting exit screening and travel restriction in countries with Ebola transmission.

The CDC sent teams of public health experts to West Africa to assist with response efforts, including surveillance, contact tracing, data management, laboratory testing, and health education; the CDC continues to send experts to the affected countries. The CDC has deployed a total of 2,110 teams since the 2014 outbreak occurred, the largest CDC response in its history.

Source: www.cdc.gov/vhf/ebola/outbreaks/2014-west-africa/what-cdc-is-doing.html

What Is Public Health?

To define *public health*, we must first define *health*. The WHO defines health as "a state of complete physical, mental and social well-being and not merely the absence of disease or infirmity" (http://www.who.int/en/). According to this definition, being healthy is more than just not being sick. It is a state of well-being in our bodies, our minds, and our lives. Keeping this definition in mind, what happens when we place the word *public* in front of the word *health*? Public in this sense implies the government has primary responsibility for the social good of health, just as it does in public education. Public health, therefore, involves the well-being of all of us as we live together in neighborhoods, communities, states, and countries. It is anything and everything that relates to helping us collectively experience "a state of complete physical, mental and social well-being." It touches nearly every aspect of our lives. The large-scale goals of public health are to protect, promote, and restore health and to reduce the premature death

curative medical care
Medical care that helps cure an already ill or infected person.

prevention efforts
Health programs and behaviors that prevent illness from occurring.

block grants Money granted by the national government to a state government with few restrictions on its spending. This can be contrasted with a categorical grant, which has strict and specific provisions on the way it is to be spent.

case A term used in health statistics to refer to each person who has a disease.

and discomfort caused by disease. In short, the goal of public health is to protect the community from the hazards of group life.

Unlike **curative medical care**, which focuses on making us feel better when we are already ill, public health focuses on **prevention efforts** to keep us from getting sick in the first place. Because it focuses on prevention, public health has the power to impact the policies and laws that help us have a healthier society. It helps promote well-being on a societal level and often global level, and it makes the world a better place for all of us.

Public health can be seen in our everyday lives in things as simple as the crosswalk lines on a street that allow us to cross a roadway without getting hit by a car or the laws requiring construction workers to wear hard hats so that they are not injured by falling construction debris. It is also recognizable in state and nation-wide campaigns to reduce smoking, heart disease, and cancer. Public health is actualized by activities such as nurses providing free immunizations to low-income children and police officers enforcing laws around seat belt and helmet use.

Most important, public health is the way a society reaches out to protect the health of its most vulnerable members. Using a system of **block grants** and specific public health initiatives, public health programs nationwide provide medical care for the elderly, substance abuse recovery programs, nutritional help for low-income women and infants, free dental care for children, medical care for the homeless, and so much more.

Public health is a wonderful idea, but does it really matter? Shouldn't it be enough for each of us just to take care of ourselves? Although our individual efforts to stay healthy do, in one sense, help us create a healthy community, some things require collective, organized efforts. For example, laws are needed to govern sanitation, waste disposal, food safety, and water purity. The quality of these services can affect an entire community. In the absence of public health efforts, it is easier for disease to spread and make more people ill.

Widespread illness affects not only people but also communities and economies. Think for a moment about the devastating effect of HIV infection in sub-Saharan Africa today. Of the 35 million AIDS **cases** (each case represents one person) worldwide in 2013, the vast majority are in this one region (http://www.unaids.org/en/dataanalysis/datatools/aidsinfo). Young adults in the prime of life are dying. Not only are families devastated and children orphaned, but large sections of the population are not working because of premature death and illness. When people can't work, food is not grown, resulting in starvation, which leads to further problems, and the situation only worsens. Although some health programs are operating in Africa, they are clearly overwhelmed by the demands on their limited resources. The lack of a strong public health system can be the downfall of a society. Public health does more than keep us healthy; it makes civilization possible.

The History of Public Health

Public health is not a completely new concept in human society. Humans have tried to promote community health in a variety of ways at different points in history. One of the earliest ways was through sanitation efforts. The ancient city of Mojenjo Daro in northern India, built over 4,000 years ago, had paved streets covering sewers that drained waste from bathrooms in residential homes. The classical era of the Greek and Roman civilizations also saw the creation of bathhouses to promote cleanliness and the building of drainage canals (Fairbanks and Wiese 1997). Early versions of **quarantine** were instituted in the Middle Ages (and earlier) when persons infected with leprosy were placed in leper colonies outside town limits in an effort to keep the disease from spreading.

quarantine Forced isolation of a person to prevent a disease from spreading.

In the United States, public health efforts gained strength as the nation grew toward independence in the 1700s. Several key events helped shape public health. Some of the first efforts of organized action to protect community health were the creation of boards of health. These early boards of health were often created in response to an **epidemic** (Turnock 2011). For example, in 1793, a terrible epidemic of yellow fever broke out in Philadelphia, then the nation's capital. The epidemic was so devastating that it prompted not only the transfer of the national capital to Washington but also the establishment of Philadelphia's first board of health that same year.

epidemic A term used to describe a disease that is widespread in a population.

The National Institutes of Health (NIH) traces its roots to 1887, when a one-room laboratory was created within the Marine Hospital Service (MHS), predecessor agency to the U.S. Public Health Service (PHS). The MHS had been established in 1798 to provide for the medical care of merchant seamen. One clerk in the Treasury Department collected 20 cents per month from the wages of each seaman to cover costs at a series of contract hospitals. In the 1880s, Congress had charged the MHS with examining passengers on arriving ships for clinical signs of infectious diseases, especially for the dreaded diseases such as cholera and yellow fever, in order to prevent epidemics. During the 1870s and 1880s, moreover, scientists in Europe presented compelling evidence that microscopic organisms were the causes of several infectious diseases. In 1884, for example, Koch described a comma-shaped bacterium as the cause of cholera. Officials of the MHS followed these developments with great interest. In 1887, they authorized Joseph J. Kinyoun, a young MHS physician trained in the new bacteriological methods, to set up a one-room laboratory in the Marine Hospital at Stapleton, Staten Island, New York. Kinyoun called this facility a "laboratory of hygiene" in imitation of German facilities and to indicate that the laboratory's purpose was to serve the public's health. Within a few months, Kinyoun had identified the cholera bacillus in suspicious cases and used his Zeiss microscope to demonstrate it to his colleagues as confirmation of their clinical diagnoses. "As the symptoms . . . were by no means well defined," he wrote, "the examinations were confirmatory evidence of the value of bacteria cultivation as a means of positive diagnosis" (NIH n.d.).

One of the key events to shape public health in America was the signing of the Act for the Relief of Sick and Disabled Seamen by President John Adams in 1798 (see Table 10.1). The act provided for a tax of 20 cents a month on the salary of sailors. The funds were used to build and staff hospitals to care for sailors. Over time, this system of hospitals and the person appointed to oversee it became the government body on which we rely today to protect our nation's health: the U.S. Public Health Service, headed by the Surgeon General (Fairbanks and Wiese 1998).

Table 10.1	*Abbreviated Historical Development—National Institutes of Health*
1798	President John Adams signed "an Act for the relief of sick and disabled Seamen," which led to the establishment of the Marine Hospital Service.
1803	The first permanent Marine Hospital authorized to be built in Boston, Massachusetts.
1836	Library of the Office of Surgeon General of the Army established.
1870	President Grant signed a law establishing a "Bureau of the U.S. Marine Hospital Service," Treasury Department, which created central control over the hospitals, and a Supervising Surgeon (later Surgeon General).
1887	Laboratory of Hygiene established at Marine Hospital, Staten Island, New York, for research in cholera and other infectious diseases.
1891	Rocky Mountain Spotted Fever Laboratory established in Hamilton, Montana, as field station of Public Health Service.
1922	Congress authorized National Cancer Institute (NCI) and the awarding of research grants. Rocky Mountain Laboratory became part of NIH.
1949	Mental Hygiene Program of Public Health Service transferred to NIH and expanded to become National Institute of Mental Health.
1950	"Omnibus Medical Research Act" authorized the establishment of the National Institute of Neurological Diseases and Blindness and the National Institute of Arthritis and Metabolic Diseases, and the latter absorbed the Experimental Biology and Medicine Institute.
1957	The Center for Aging Research established.
1961	The Center for Research in Child Health established in Division of General Medical Sciences.
1964	Division of Computer Research and Technology established.
1966	Division of Environmental Health Sciences created.
1970	National Institute on Aging created.
1990	National Center for Research Resources was created by consolidating the Division of Research Services and the Division of Research Resources.
1991	National Center for Medical Rehabilitation Research established within the National Institute of Child Health and Human Development.
1992	National Institute on Alcohol Abuse and Alcoholism, National Institute on Drug Abuse, and National Institute of Mental Health were transferred to NIH from the Alcohol, Drug Abuse, and Mental Health Administration.
1993	National Center for Nursing Research was retitled as the National Institute of Nursing Research.
1994	The Dietary Supplement Health and Education Act of 1993 mandated establishment of an Office of Dietary Supplements within NIH to conduct and coordinate NIH research relating to dietary supplements and the extent to which their use reduces the risk of certain diseases.
2000 to present	The international Human Genome Project public consortium—funded by NIH, the Department of Energy (DOE), and others—assembled a working draft of the sequence of the human genome.
2003	The International Human Genome Sequencing Consortium, led in the United States by the National Human Genome Research Institute and the DOE, completed the Human Genome Project.

The complete genetic blueprint of *Bacillus anthracis*—the microbe that gained notoriety during the 2001 anthrax mail attacks—has been completed by NIAID-funded researchers. |

Table 10.1	(*continued*)
	President George W. Bush visits NIH on Feb. 3 to unveil Project BioShield, a $6 billion, 10-year effort to protect the public from various weapons of bioterrorism.
2004	NIH opens the Mark O. Hatfield Clinical Research Center, a 240-bed successor to the NIH Clinical Center, which opened in 1953.
2008	Through legislation enacted by Congress, NICHD was renamed the Eunice Kennedy Shriver National Institute of Child Health and Human Development at the institute's 45th anniversary celebration. In the early 1960s, Shriver persuaded her brother, President John F. Kennedy, to include the proposal for an NIH institute focusing on child health and human development in his first health message to Congress. NICHD was then established in 1963.
2010	President Obama signed the Patient Protection and Affordable Care Act.
2013	Antimalarial drug deemed safe for human use.
2014	The John Edward Porter Center for Neuroscience was opened.

Source: http://www.nih.gov/about/almanac/historical/chronology_of_events.htm

In 1850, Lemuel Shattuck published the *Report of the Sanitary Commission of Massachusetts*. It outlined the existing and future public health needs for that state and became America's blueprint for the development of public health systems. Shattuck's report called for the establishment of state and local health departments to engage in sanitary inspections, **communicable disease** control, food sanitation, vital statistics, and services for infants and children. Although it took several decades for his ideas to catch on, Massachusetts established the first state health department in 1869. By 1900, there were 40 such state health departments (CDC 1999a). The public health system was expanded considerably in the period just after the great influenza epidemic in 1918 (Berry 2004). Today, every state has a health department and a public health laboratory.

communicable disease A disease that spreads from person to person; another term for infectious disease.

Key Public Health Functions

In 1988, the Institute of Medicine released a report called *The Future of Public Health* that outlined these three key functions of public health: assessment of the health of the community, policy development, and assurance of the public health. **Assessment** means determining the health needs of the community by surveying disease incidence and prevalence, identifying needs, analyzing why health outcomes are not met, collecting and interpreting data, monitoring health trends research, and evaluating outcomes.

Policy development is the collective decision about what actions are most appropriate for the health of the state or nation. **Assurance** is making sure that the necessary actions are actually taken. To carry out these three functions, information is needed. Public health officials engage in three key activities to satisfy this need: epidemiology, surveillance, and monitoring. These activities provide them with the information they need to assess and ensure a community's health and to make policy decisions.

assessment The process of determining the health needs of a community.

policy development The process of making a collective decision about what needs to be done to protect the community's health.

assurance The process of making sure that correct actions are taken to protect community health.

epidemiology The study of the nature, cause, control, and determinants of the frequency of disease, disability, and death in human populations. Also the study of the history of a disease and its distribution throughout a society (public health).

Epidemiology is the study of the history of a disease and its distribution throughout a society. It permits understanding and rational decision making regarding actions that need to be taken. Epidemiologists investigate where a disease outbreak occurred, who it affected, and how and when. Popularized recently as "disease detectives," epidemiologists help determine not only where a disease came from but also how to protect people from it. For example, in 1993 in the state of Washington, 477 people became ill from *Escherichia coli*, a deadly bacterium that causes severe intestinal problems and sometimes death. Epidemiologists kept track of who had the disease. They investigated what activities the infected persons had engaged in up to the time when they got sick. Their research led them to a local fast-food restaurant that had been undercooking ground beef. Thanks to epidemiologists, the cause of the problem was discovered and further illness prevented. To learn more about the career of epidemiology, see the Career Profile.

surveillance The continuous search for and documentation of disease in public health.

The term *surveillance* is used to describe the actions of police as they watch a suspect and take note of what takes place. Similarly, in public health, **surveillance** refers to the continuous search for and documentation of disease. If public health departments were not always on the lookout for new diseases or outbreaks of disease, diseases could run rampant. Surveillance keeps track of all kinds of things, from sexually transmitted infections, to episodes of violence, to the number of cases of the flu.

monitoring The regular review of disease data to determine changes in disease levels.

Monitoring refers to the use of surveillance data to determine changes in the number of infected persons so that the appropriate action can be taken when the infection rate gets too high. Monitoring helps answer questions about whether or not there is more or less of a particular disease present now than in the past.

Several basic measurements can help us understand the information uncovered through surveillance and monitoring activities. Often you hear these terms used in the news or in reports about a current health concern. These measurements are used to create a picture of how a disease is affecting society. Table 10.2 lists some key public health terms.

Table 10.2	*Key Terms in Public Health Measurement*
Incidence	Number of new cases of a disease or event such as a motor vehicle accident in a specific population.
Morbidity	Number of cases of a specific disease in a specific period of time per unit of population, usually expressed as a number per 1,000.
Mortality rates	Number of people who have died from a given disease or event. These rates are collected and analyzed from death certificates. *Morbidity and Mortality Weekly Report* is published by the CDC and reports illness and death rates for a variety of diseases.
Prevalence	Total number of infected/affected people (cases) over a given period of time.
Relative risk	How an individual's risk may change relevant to a specific factor (e.g., a smoker has a higher relative risk of getting lung cancer than a person who does not smoke).
Risk	Likelihood that someone will become infected/affected.

Where do the data for surveillance and monitoring come from? State health departments are required by law to report on cases of specific diseases or conditions. Some of this data, such as the number of persons infected with a particular disease, are collected for statistical purposes and to alert health authorities to a possible epidemic. Other conditions, such as child abuse, are reported because it allows someone to intervene in the situation and ideally prevent any further abuse from occurring. Whenever health or social service providers come across one of these conditions or diseases, they are required to report the information to the state. This information can be reported confidentially. For example, although the number of people infected with HIV is reported to the state, their names are not. As of 2012, 91 diseases had to be reported at the national level, including HIV, cholera, rabies, sexually transmitted infections, tuberculosis, hepatitis, and anthrax exposure (see Table 10.3).

Table 10.3	*Infectious Diseases Designated as Notifiable at the National Level During 2012*

Anthrax
Arboviral diseases, neuroinvasive and
   nonneuroinvasive
Babesiosis
Botulism: foodborne, infant, other (wound and
   unspecified)
Brucellosis
California serogroup viruses
  Eastern equine encephalitis virus
  Powassan virus
  St. Louis encephalitis virus
  West Nile virus
  Western equine encephalitis virus
Chancroid
Chlamydia trachomatis infection
Cholera toxigenic *Vibrio cholerae* 01 or 0139
Coccidioidomycosis
Crimean-Congo hemorrhagic fever virus
Cryptosporidiosis[†]
Cyclosporiasis
Dengue virus infections
Dengue fever
Dengue hemorrhagic fever
Dengue shock syndrome
Diphtheria
Ebola virus
Ehrlichiosis/Anaplasmosis
  Ehrlichia chaffeensis
  Ehrlichia ewingii
  Anaplasma phagocytophilum
  Undetermined human ehrlichiosis/anaplasmosis
Giardiasis
Gonorrhea

Haemophilus influenzae, invasive disease
Hansen disease (leprosy)
Hantavirus pulmonary syndrome
Hemolytic uremic syndrome, post-diarrheal
Hepatitis, viral
Hepatitis A, acute[†]
Hepatitis B, acute[†]
Hepatitis B virus, perinatal infection
Hepatitis B, chronic[†]
Hepatitis C, acute[†]
Hepatitis C, past or present[†]
Human Immunodeficiency Virus (HIV) infection
  diagnosis[§]
Influenza-associated pediatric mortality
Invasive pneumococcal disease
Lassa virus
Legionellosis
Listeriosis
Lujo virus
Lyme disease
Malaria
Marburg virus
Measles
Meningococcal disease
Mumps[†]
New World arenaviruses (Guanarito, Lujo,
  Machupo, Junin, and Sabia viruses)
Novel influenza A virus infections
Pertussis
Plague
Poliomyelitis, paralytic
Poliovirus infection, nonparalytic
Psittacosis

(continued)

Table 10.3 *(continued)*	
Q fever	Tetanus
Acute	Toxic-shock syndrome (other than
Chronic	streptococcal)
Rabies	Trichinellosis
Animal	Tuberculosis
Human	Tularemia
Rubella	Typhoid fever
Rubella, congenital syndrome	Vancomycin-intermediate *Staphylococcus aureus*
Salmonellosis†	(VISA) infection
Severe acute respiratory syndrome-associated	Vancomycin-resistant *Staphylococcus aureus*
coronavirus (SARS-CoV) disease	(VRSA) infection
Shiga toxin-producing *Escherichia coli* (STEC)	Varicella (morbidity)
Shigellosis†	Varicella (mortality)
Smallpox	Vibriosis†
Spotted fever rickettsiosis	Any species of the family Vibrionaceae, other than
Streptococcal toxic-shock syndrome	toxigenic *Vibrio cholerae* 01 or 0139
Syphilis	Viral hemorrhagic fever
Syphilis, congenital	Yellow fever

*This list reflects position statements approved in 2011 by the Council of State and Territorial Epidemiologists (CSTE) for national surveillance, which were implemented in January 2012. No additions or deletions of diseases or conditions were made to the list of nationally notifiable infectious diseases. National surveillance case definitions for these diseases and conditions are available at http://wwwn.cdc.gov/nndss/.

†The year 2012 reflects a modified surveillance case definition for this condition, per approved 2011 CSTE position statements.

§AIDS has been reclassified as HIV stage III.

Source: CDC 2014.

Career Profile: Epidemiologist

Epidemiologists are sometimes called "disease detectives." Like any good detective, their primary duty is to carry out investigations, in this case of a disease. They study where a disease outbreak occurred, who it affected, and how and when. They examine the relationships among various factors such as lifestyle, environment, person-to-person contact, and geography. They collect information from people using surveys and interviews. They also look at existing health information such as local disease statistics or insurance claims information.

Epidemiologists can work in health departments, laboratories, hospitals, and government agencies, such as the CDC. Because disease outbreaks can occur anywhere at any time, some epidemiologists travel the nation, or even the world, for their investigations.

Other epidemiologists investigate disease outbreaks closer to home. When not investigating a disease, epidemiologists work at their computers cataloging all the information they have collected.

The conclusions reached by epidemiologists and the data they collect are important in several ways. First, in determining how a disease is spread, epidemiologists can make recommendations about how to avoid further infections. Second, their conclusions can help boards of health and health departments develop policies to protect the community's health. Without the work of epidemiologists, our understanding of diseases and how they pass from person to person would be severely limited. Thanks to epidemiologists, our path to health gets clearer, and a little bit easier, all the time.

Role of Government in Public Health

The government plays a key role in ensuring the public's health. Government in action can be seen at the local (county, neighborhood), state, and federal levels. Prior to the Great Depression (1929–41), U.S. citizens did not think the federal government should intervene in people's health. Health is not a power granted to the federal government in the Constitution. Therefore, individuals, with some help from the state government, took care of their health themselves. But the situation was so desperate during the Great Depression that the federal government was expected to take action (Turnock 2011).

Since then, the federal government's role in health has expanded. Two sections of the Constitution have been interpreted as allowing the federal government to intervene in the nation's health. The first is the ability to tax people to provide for the "general welfare." This allows for the collection of money to be used in support of health programs. In fact, today the government's main role in public health is financial support of public health programs.

Second, the federal government has the ability to regulate commerce. Only the government can enforce policies that limit the personal and property rights of individuals or businesses. This power allows for the regulation of restaurants, sewage and water companies, product and drug safety, and other businesses that sell products to consumers.

Federal Government

Public health at the federal level is represented by numerous agencies, each dedicated to a specific aspect of the public's health. The Department of Health and Human Services (DHHS) is the U.S. government's principal department protecting the health of the nation. Here is a list of some of these key agencies and their responsibilities:

- The Food and Drug Administration (FDA) ensures the safety of foods, cosmetics, and medications.
- The CDC works with state health departments and other community organizations to monitor disease, help prevent outbreaks, maintain national health statistics, and operate disease-prevention and health-promotion programs.
- The Health Resources and Services Administration (HRSA) provides access to health care services for low-income and uninsured people or for people who live in areas where health care is not easily available. In 2013, HRSA-funded health care centers provided medical care for more than 21.7 million people in 1,202 health centers across the nation (http://bphc.hrsa.gov/uds/datacenter.aspx).
- The Centers for Medicare & Medicaid Services (CMS) provides health care insurance through third-party carriers for about one in every four

Americans. Medicare provides insurance for more than 43 million elderly and persons with disabilities (www.cms.gov). Medicaid covers low-income persons, including children. The Affordable Care Act encourages states to expand coverage (see Chapter 4 for a more detailed discussion).

■ The Substance Abuse and Mental Health Services Administration (SAMHSA) works to improve the availability and quality of substance abuse prevention, addiction treatment, and mental health services. Funding from SAMSHA helps millions of Americans with serious substance abuse problems or mental health problems (www.samhsa.gov).

As mentioned earlier in the chapter, public health is the way a society cares for its most vulnerable citizens. The government's financial involvement is clearly crucial to this effort. Without this support, literally millions of individuals would be without adequate medical care. Our ability to control disease would be severely hampered. A government's investment in public health is a symbol of how much it supports and cares for its citizens.

State Government

At the state level, there are two kinds of public health bodies: boards of health and state health departments. Boards of health are the policymaking bodies for a state's Department of Health. States that do not have boards of health have other mechanisms to make policy. They have the power to adopt and amend rules and regulations and to make recommendations. State health departments are charged with promoting the public's health and implementing public health laws. States regulate things like newborn screening. Most states require PKU and other genetic disorders screening. Many have provisions for treating these defects with special formulas and other necessary interventions through the Health Departments.

Additional responsibilities of state departments of health include

■ Carrying out national and state mandates designed to protect health
■ Managing environmental education and personal health services
■ Collecting, analyzing, and disseminating information on threats to the community's health
■ Responding to statewide health crises such as hepatitis and flu outbreaks
■ Setting policies and standards for health care and medical professionals
■ Conducting inspections of restaurants and factories
■ Conducting the planning and evaluation of health programs

There are two models of a state health department. In most states, the health department is a freestanding agency that reports directly to the state governor. In other states, the health department is part of a larger institution, such as the state's Department of Health and Human Services. Under the Affordable Care

Act, state health departments have taken on increased responsibilities for outreach and enrollment (http://www.healthcare.gov/).

In addition, licensing and regulatory boards help protect the public's health by ensuring that health care professionals and others, such as food handlers, are held to basic standards of care, cleanliness, and safety. For example, state health inspectors evaluate whether or not laboratories are using proper techniques, if restaurants have adequate food safety efforts, or if a factory has strong enough pollution control measures. As you read in the chapters about health professionals, licensing boards assure consumers that their health or service professionals have been tested and trained on specific knowledge. Not only are health professionals licensed, but in many states so are service personnel such as food handlers and cosmeticians.

Local Health Departments

Local health departments can serve an individual county, city, or region. They are responsible for the delivery of services mandated by the state or by local statute. They can be independent or part of a state department of health.

The most common programs and services include adult and child immunizations, communicable disease control, community assessment, community education, environmental health services, epidemiology and surveillance, food safety, restaurant inspections, and tuberculosis testing. These local agencies rarely provide direct medical care. Some of these responsibilities have shifted due to the increase in coverage for preventive services under the Affordable Care Act (www.naccho.org/topics/healthreform/). Because state government has so many administrative, legal, and inspection responsibilities, it is important to have local health systems that can provide more direct service to community members.

Other Public Health Partners

Public health is not solely in the hands of the government. Organizations like the Red Cross, March of Dimes, and the American Cancer Society play an important role. In addition, smaller local social service organizations are able to work directly with the community members whose health they want to protect. These may be not-for-profit organizations or community-based organizations. They provide services in their local communities for specific populations and for one or two targeted health problems. For example, an organization could choose to help inner-city homeless youth or young women with substance abuse problems. **Foundations** are a particular kind of not-for-profit organization. They raise funds to support a cause of their choice and then distribute the funding to other community-based organizations in support of their work.

The importance of these nongovernmental partners cannot be underestimated. In particular, community-based organizations often go directly to the

foundation A type of not-for-profit organization that raises money and then distributes it to other organizations in support of their programs.

person needing services. Sometimes this means visiting people in their homes or finding them in parks or on the street. Thus many people who might not make it to the health department receive the help they need. By specializing in a specific health issue, these organizations can also provide expert advice to their patrons. Nongovernmental efforts help complete and strengthen the public health system.

Past Successes and Future Challenges

According to the CDC, the life expectancy of persons living in the United States has increased by 30 years since 1900; 25 years of this gain are attributable to successful public health interventions. Although the successes of public health are many, the CDC selected key program areas as having the most impact on lowering death rates and decreasing illness and disability in the United States (CDC 1999b). These 10 great achievements are related to the following areas:

1. Vaccination: The development of vaccines and vaccination campaigns has led to decreased incidences of many illnesses such as diphtheria. Also, vaccinations have eradicated diseases such as smallpox and, in the Western Hemisphere, polio.
2. Safer workplaces: New safety standards in industries such as mining, construction, manufacturing, and transportation have led to a 40 percent reduction in the rate of job-related injuries.
3. Healthier mothers and babies: Improvements in hygiene, nutrition, and availability of antibiotics; greater access to health care; and technological advances have helped reduce infant and maternal mortality.

infectious disease A disease that can spread from person to person (versus a genetic disease or a disease that is not contagious).

4. Control of **infectious diseases**: Improved sanitation and clean water have helped control many diseases such as cholera and typhoid. Also, new medications have helped control the spread of diseases like tuberculosis and sexually transmitted infections.
5. Coronary heart disease and stroke prevention programs: Education regarding smoking cessation, blood pressure control, and the importance of early detection has led to a 51 percent decrease in death rates since 1972.
6. Safer and healthier foods: The identification of essential nutrients and food fortification programs (e.g., adding iodine to salt or vitamin D to milk) have nearly eliminated diseases such as rickets and goiter.
7. Family planning: Access to family planning has provided health benefits such as smaller family sizes and longer intervals between the births of children. In addition, the use of barrier contraceptives (condoms) has helped prevent unwanted pregnancies and the transmission of HIV and other sexually transmitted diseases.

Medical Reserve Corps

The Medical Reserve Corps (MRC) was founded after President Bush's 2002 State of the Union Address, in which he asked all Americans to volunteer in support of their country. It is a partner program with Citizen Corps, a national network of volunteers dedicated to ensuring hometown security. The U.S. Surgeon General assigns MRC units specific areas to target that strengthen the public health infrastructure of their communities each year. These reflect the priorities for the health of individuals, and the nation as a whole. The goal, in addition to providing well-trained volunteers in an emergency, is to improve health literacy, and in support of this, he wants us to work toward increasing disease prevention, eliminating health disparities, and improving public health preparedness. Units are community based and function as a way to locally organize and utilize volunteers who want to donate their time and expertise to prepare for and respond to emergencies and promote healthy living throughout the year. MRC volunteers supplement existing emergency and public health resources.

MRC volunteers include medical and public health professionals such as physicians, nurses, pharmacists, dentists, veterinarians, and epidemiologists. Many community members—interpreters, chaplains, office workers, legal advisors, and others—fill key support positions.

MRC volunteers can also choose to support communities in need nationwide. When the Southeast was battered by hurricanes in 2004, MRC volunteers in the affected areas and beyond helped communities by filling in at local hospitals, assisting their neighbors at local shelters, and providing first aid to those injured by the storms. During this 2-month period, more than 30 MRC units worked as part of the relief efforts, including those whose volunteers were called in from across the country to assist the American Red Cross (ARC) and the Federal Emergency Management Agency (FEMA).

During the 2012 hurricane season, Hurricane Sandy, the largest hurricane ever to impact the United States, affected 24 states. MRC members provided support for ARC health services, mental health, and shelter operations. MRC members also supported the HHS response and recovery efforts by staffing special needs shelters, community health centers, and health clinics and by assisting health assessment teams in those states. More than 155 MRC units were deployed outside their local jurisdiction on optional missions to the disaster-affected areas with their state agencies, the ARC, and HHS; the units provided more than 36,000 hours of volunteer service to those affected by Hurricane Sandy. During the 2009 flu pandemic, volunteers set up vaccination stations in schools, public meeting places, and fire stations. The McMinnville, Oregon, MRC unit vaccinated more than 10,000 at-risk schoolchildren and adults within a 4-week period.

MRC volunteers attend training sessions and must be certified in Incident Command Strategy to facilitate the integration of the volunteers with Emergency Response teams to avoid some of the confusion found in early large-scale disasters.

Sources: http://www.medicalreservecorps.gov/; Photo: http://www.medicalreservecorps.gov/image/PhotoGallery/Training/ExerSep09-006.jpg

8. Motor vehicle safety: Improvements in both car and highway design and successful education programs to change personal behavior (e.g., wearing seat belts, helmets, not drinking and driving) have led to large reductions in vehicle-related deaths.

9. Fluoridation of drinking water: Since 1945, fluoride has been added to drinking water and has helped to reduce tooth decay in children (40 percent to 70 percent) and tooth loss in adults (40 percent to 60 percent).

10. Recognition of tobacco as a health hazard: Antismoking campaigns have helped prevent initiation of tobacco use, promoted quitting, and reduced environmental tobacco smoke. The prevalence of smoking among adults has decreased, and millions of smoking-related deaths have been prevented.

Even with all these successes, there remains much work to be done. What are the new challenges for public health in the next 100 years? Public health must meet several new challenges in the future, such as changing patterns of disease, increasing numbers of chronic conditions, new and emerging infections, injuries, violence, and curable genetic diseases (Turnock 2011). Diseases once thought under control, like tuberculosis, are making a comeback because of global travel into and out of countries where these diseases are common and in specific populations such as those with compromised immune systems. Antibiotics, one of our most powerful weapons in the fight against disease, are becoming increasingly ineffective as many bacteria become **drug resistant** (i.e., the bacteria are no longer killed by the antibiotic). Global travel allows for the quick spread of disease across borders. The United States faces a range of wholly preventable diseases and conditions that have reached epidemic proportions, such as HIV/AIDS, obesity, and stress-related conditions. In the next 100 years, public health must continue to adapt and expand its capacity to address these new health concerns.

drug resistant The term used to describe when a disease or bacteria is not affected or stopped by the use of common antibiotics and other drugs.

Career Profile: Environmental Health Specialist (EHS)

This career combines science, detective work, and public service. It can be a stepping-stone to a career in epidemiology or a stand-alone career in a local or state public health department. It could lead to a position as a commissioned officer in the U.S. Public Health Service Commissioned Corps or military.

The role of the EHS is to prevent and control infectious disease by enforcing health and safety standards related to food, water, septic, and consumer product safety. EHSs also track disease through public health surveillance tools. They collect, analyze, and interpret data about health events such as childhood diseases or outbreaks of foodborne illness and health risks resulting from disasters like floods and extreme weather.

On the job the EHS might be found inspecting restaurants, hotels, swimming pools, water sources, day care facilities, food processing plants, and schools to ensure health standards are being met. The EHS collects data on disease outbreaks and environmental incidents such as chemical spills, pesticide contamination, and contamination of water sources. EHSs frequently work for public agencies such as county health departments and state agencies such as the Department of Agriculture or the Department of Environmental Quality.

Entry-level positions require a bachelor's degree, either in public health or in biology, microbiology, or chemistry. Most states require 1 to 2 years of internship, as well as a certification exam. There is a national certification board. An EHS can expect to earn $46,000. With experience, salaries grow to the $100,000 range. State and federal employees usually have good benefit packages.

A related field is wastewater specialist. The job focuses on wastewater systems such as septic. This specialist could analyze soil data as part of the design and installation of a system that uses soil as part of the disposal process. A bachelor's degree in soil science and 2 years of experience under a certified wastewater specialist are required, or a master's with 1 year of experience. A certification exam is also required for employment.

Summary

In this chapter, you read about the history of public health both globally and in the United States. Public health refers to any and all organized and collaborative efforts that are undertaken with the goal of protecting community health. The basic public health activities are assessment of the health of the community, policy development, and assurance of the public health. Health professionals who study disease and monitor key data perform these activities. The government is involved at the federal, state, and local levels to carry out these activities. Foundations and other private partners also play a role in ensuring the nation's health.

Questions for Review

1. Define public health.
2. List the three key functions of public health.
3. Name a public health agency, and define its role.
4. Define incidence, morbidity, and mortality rate.
5. List one public health achievement.
6. See the profile at the beginning of the chapter. What public health measures were taken to protect the United States from Ebola? Were they effective?

7. Compare and contrast the public health response to Ebola and H1N1 flu epidemics.
8. Explain what an epidemiologist does to help control disease.

Questions for Discussion

1. What do you think the role of the federal government should be in public health? Are public health efforts worth all the tax dollars you pay for them?
2. If public health is really so successful, why are people still getting sick and engaging in behaviors that are bad for their health?
3. What do you think are the most important problems for public health to address today?
4. Why do we need so many types of health departments at the federal, state, and local levels? Does public health help create too much of a government bureaucracy? Why, or why not? Does it matter?
5. Is it more important for the government to invest in curative medical care or in prevention efforts? What are the benefits and drawbacks of each?
6. Would you volunteer for the Medical Reserve Corps in your community? Why? Why not?

Chapter References

Berry, J. 2004. *The great influenza: The epic story of the deadliest plague in history.* London: Penguin Books.

Centers for Disease Control and Prevention (CDC). September 19, 2014. Summary of notifiable diseases, 2012. *Mortality and Morbidity Weekly Report* 61(53).

_____. 1999a. Achievements in public health, 1900–1999: Changes in the public health system. *Mortality and Morbidity Weekly Report* 48(50): 1141–47.

_____. 1999b. Ten great public health achievements: United States 1900–1999. *Mortality and Morbidity Weekly Report* 48(12): 21–243.

Centers for Disease Control and Prevention (http://www.cdc.gov).

Fairbanks, J., and W. Wiese. 1997. *The public health primer.* Thousand Oaks, CA: Sage.

http://bphc.hrsa.gov/uds/datacenter.aspx.

HealthCare.gov (http://www.healthcare.gov/).

Medical Reserve Corps (http://www.medicalreservecorps.gov/).

National Institutes of Health (NIH) (http://www.nih.gov/about/almanac/historical/chronology_of_events.htm).

National Institutes of Health (NIH). *A short history of the National Institutes of Health.* (http://www.history.nih.gov/exhibits/history).

Turnock, B. 2011. *Public health: What it is and how it works.* 5th ed. Burlington, MA: Jones and Bartlett Learning.

UNAIDS: The Joint United Nations Programme on HIV/AIDS (www.unaids.org).

World Health Organization (http://www.who.int/en/).

For Additional Information

Centers for Disease Control and Prevention, Emergency Preparedness and Response (http://www.bt.cdc.gov/).

International Network for the History of Public Health (http://www.liu.se/tema/inhph/).

Mullan, F. 1989. *Plagues and politics: The story of the United States public health service.* New York: Basic Books.

State and Local Government on the Net (http://www.statelocalgov.net/).

11

Medical Technology, Pharmaceuticals, and Pharmacological Research

Learning Objectives

After reading this chapter, you should be able to:

1. Define medical technology.
2. Discuss the impact of medical technology on modern health care.
3. Identify the ethical issues in new technologies.
4. Discuss the size and scope of the pharmaceutical industry.
5. Explain how a new prescription drug gets to market.
6. Identify how new prescription drugs are marketed.
7. Discuss the ethical issues in pharmaceuticals.

Stem Cells for the Future Treatment of Parkinson's Disease

Parkinson's disease (PD) is a neurodegenerative disorder that affects more than 2 percent of the population older than 65 years. PD is caused by a progressive degeneration and loss of dopamine (DA)-producing neurons, which leads to tremor, rigidity, and hypokinesia (abnormally decreased mobility). It is thought that PD may be the first disease to be amenable to treatment using stem cell transplantation. Factors that support this idea include the knowledge of the specific cell type (DA neurons) needed to relieve the symptoms of the disease. In addition, several laboratories have been successful in developing methods to induce embryonic stem cells to differentiate into cells with many of the functions of DA neurons.

In a recent study, scientists directed mouse embryonic stem cells to differentiate into DA neurons by introducing the gene Nurr1. When transplanted into the brains of a rat model of PD, these stem cell–derived DA neurons reinnervated the brains of the rat Parkinson model, released dopamine, and improved motor function.

Regarding human stem cell therapy, scientists are developing a number of strategies for producing dopamine neurons from human stem cells in the laboratory for transplantation into humans with PD. The successful generation of an unlimited supply of dopamine neurons could make neurotransplantation widely available for Parkinson's patients at some point in the future.

Source: http://stemcells.nih.gov/info/basics/

Introduction

technology The application of knowledge based on inventions, innovations, and discoveries in science.

medical technology Therapeutic and diagnostic devices used to prevent, treat, diagnose, and assist patients medically. The X-ray machine is an example of medical technology.

pharmaceuticals Bioactive agents in the human body for therapeutic purposes (e.g., antibiotics).

Medical technology and pharmaceuticals are an increasingly important and expensive part of modern health care. **Technology** is the application of knowledge based on inventions, innovations, and discoveries in science. Table 11.1 presents a picture of technological advances in health care from the 1800s to the present. Just as Pasteur's proof that microorganisms cause disease fundamentally changed the ways physicians treated patients in the 19th century, today's technological advances have changed who treats patients, how health care professionals are trained, how they interact with patients, and health care economics.

This chapter addresses advances in medical technology and in the pharmaceutical industry. **Medical technology** in this chapter means those therapeutic and diagnostic devices used by health professionals to prevent, treat, and diagnose illness and assist patients medically. This includes everything from ordinary items such as stethoscopes and blood pressure monitors to the latest in imaging machines and in vitro diagnostic tests. **Pharmaceuticals** are the research, production, marketing, and dispensing of agents (drugs, genes, molecules, etc.) that are bioactive in the human body for therapeutic purposes. Each of these has produced global industries and impacts the delivery of health care.

Table 11.1	*Technological Advances in Health Care*

1819	René Laennec invents the stethoscope
1846	American dentist Dr. William Morton uses ether as anesthetic
1847	Dr. James Simpson uses chloroform as anesthetic
1879	Louis Pasteur proves microorganisms cause disease
1865	Joseph Lister uses disinfectants and antiseptics during surgery to prevent infection
1892	Dimitri Ivanovski discovers viruses
1895	Wilhelm Roentgen discovers X-rays (roentgenograms)
1896	Almroth Wright develops vaccine for typhoid fever
1901	Carl Landsteiner classifies ABO blood groups
1923	Frederick Banting and Charles Best discover and use insulin to treat diabetes
1932	Sir Alexander Fleming discovers penicillin
1944	First kidney dialysis machine is developed
1952	Jonas Salk develops polio vaccine
1953	Francis Crick and James Watson describe the structure of DNA First heart-lung machine is used for open-heart surgery
1954	Joseph Murray performs first successful human kidney transplant
1960	Birth control pills are approved by the FDA
1963	Thomas Starzl performs first liver transplant
1964	James Hardy performs first lung transplant
1968	Christian Barnard performs first successful heart transplant
1975	CT (computerized axial tomography) scan is developed
1980s	Vaccines against hepatitis, herpes simplex, and chicken pox are developed with genetic engineering
1981	AIDS (acquired immune deficiency syndrome) is identified as a disease
1987	First laser surgery on human cornea
1990	First gene therapy is developed to treat disease
1990s	Rapid increase in identification of genes causing disease occurs
1995	Lasik eye surgery approved by FDA
2000	First robotic system for general laparoscopic surgery approved by FDA
2001	RNAi: RNA interference is a process to deactivate selected genes
2003	Drug-eluting stent for clogged arteries approved by FDA
2006	First vaccine to protect against cervical cancer
2008	Commercial hybrid PET/MRI scanner produced
2013	Precise proton therapy delivery systems
2015	Magnetic nanoparticles used to stop strokes
2015	Transfemoral aortic valve replacement

Sources: Bryan 1996; CDC 2009, Figure 23; and http://www.ncbi.nlm.nih.gov/pmc/articles/PMC3549771/.

Medical Technology

Medical technology is a growth area of health care, from both a business perspective and delivery perspective. According to the Annual Survey of Manufacturers, production of medical equipment and supplies was valued at $95 billion in 2013. The industry employs about 281,000 people, with a total payroll of $17 billion (U.S. Census Bureau 2013). These figures do not include some **medical devices**, including electromedical equipment such as pacemakers, MRI machines, and diagnostic medical imaging, nor does it include irradiation apparatus, such as X-ray devices or CT equipment. The surgical supplies and instruments categories account for more than 50 percent of the industry's sales, which means that every visit to an office, clinic, or hospital is impacted by the medical technology industry.

medical devices The range of medical technologies that are used for therapeutic purposes such as cardiac pacemakers and thermometers.

Medical technology is an innovative industry. The industry invests about 11 percent of sales in **research and development** (**R&D**). By comparison, the auto industry invests 4 percent, and the aerospace industry invests 3 percent. Because companies rigorously protect their investments, there is considerable patent litigation concerning medical technology.

research and development (R&D) The process of examining and bringing a product to market.

Although there continue to be advances and major breakthroughs daily, the last 20 years have seen advances in four areas that have made enormous differences in health care outcomes. These four areas are medical devices, medical imaging, minimally invasive surgery, and genetic mapping and testing.

Medical Devices

Medical devices cover a wide range of technologies from medical implants (cardiac pacemakers) to fetal or heart monitors to a simple manual blood pressure cuff. The modern hospital utilizes hundreds, perhaps thousands, of medical devices. The stock of many medical device companies is publicly traded on the New York Stock Exchange, an indication of the profitability of this segment of the health care industry.

implants Medical devices that are placed inside the human body for therapeutic purposes, such as an insulin pump or artificial knee joint.

Implants are one part of this growing medical device sector. Cardiac pacemakers are just one of many implantable devices designed to enhance or replace injured or nonfunctioning tissue. Others include bionic limbs, eyes, cochlear ear implants, nerve stimulators, medication pumps (insulin and pain medication), and whole organs such as the heart.

These devices have the potential to dramatically improve the quality of life. And once the new technology is developed, physicians and patients want to use it. This is creating a huge technology divide between the insured and uninsured populations. Those who can afford these devices experience a much improved quality of life with far less morbidity.

medical imaging Viewing the inside of the human body using a variety of techniques such as X-rays and CT scans.

Medical Imaging

Medical imaging includes a wide variety of techniques to provide visual images of the inside of the body. Nothing since the invention of the X-ray has changed medical diagnosis as much as the computer. New computer-enhanced tools allow us not only to visualize what is going on inside the body but also to watch body processes in real time. This technology will continue to advance rapidly as computer capability increases and the tools to visualize at a molecular level are developed. These new tools will improve the diagnostic ability of the physician but will come at a high economic cost.

A number of different energy sources are currently used for medical imaging. These include traditional X-rays, **CAT scans (computer axial tomography)**, ultrasound, electron beams, positrons, and magnets and radio frequencies (**magnetic resonance imaging, or MRI**). As these sources are combined with improved contrast materials and improved computer displays, the ability to diagnose abnormalities and to study the body functions will be vastly enhanced. This will in turn lead to even more sophisticated imaging than currently possible.

For example, instead of using the traditional X-ray, **electron beam computer tomography** can be used. This technology creates images using electrons instead of X-rays. Patient care is improved by reducing the time and discomfort a patient experiences being immobile and confined for a conventional CT scan. Patients and health care payers will have to decide whether the benefit outweighs the increased cost.

Minimally Invasive Surgery

Minimally invasive surgery refers to the use of fiberoptics, guided images, microwave, laser, high-intensity focused ultrasound, cryotherapy, and the newest addition—radio frequency—to do operations without the traditional open surgery. Through the use of miniature cameras, image-guided surgery now makes possible the intraorgan repair of tissue. In the past, the patient would have to undergo major open surgery with ribs, cartilage, muscle, and soft tissue being disturbed, cut, or removed. Now single or multiple scopes are inserted through small openings, and whole organs are then removed, explored, or repaired. It is even possible to perform surgery on the fetus using intrauterine technology to repair heart and spinal defects before birth.

The techniques for thermal destruction of tissue began with **electrocautery** for small-size tissue like blood vessels. The field has progressed to microwave therapy and destruction of tumors using laparoscopic techniques combined with thermal technology. Until recently, the technique could not be used for large tumors because a large mass of tissue could not be heated. The use of **radio frequency ablation (RFA)** overcame that limitation; RFA is being used safely for tumors of the liver, heart, kidney, and more (http://www.cc.nih.gov/drd/rfa/pdf/physicians.pdf).

Other forms of less-invasive surgery combine thermal, radio frequencies, and mechanical ablation with fiberoptic visualization. The recovery times have decreased from several months to days. Although the medical devices to achieve these results are very expensive, the cost in terms of patient outcome and loss of work productivity has been lowered. This leads to recommendation for some types of surgery as both therapeutic and preventative (e.g., in the case of cardiac angioplasty). Indications for surgery have changed in the light of the recent developments in less-invasive techniques.

CAT scans (computer axial tomography) Machine that visualizes the inside of the human body using a combination of X-ray technology and computerized axial tomography; results are viewed on the computer.

magnetic resonance imaging (MRI) Technology that uses electromagnetic radiation to visualize the body's soft tissues, such as the brain and spinal cord.

electron beam computer tomography Uses electron beams instead of X-rays for computerized axial tomography and also viewed on computer. Compared with the traditional CT scan, it does not require the patient to be completely still, is less enclosed, and costs more.

minimally invasive surgery Use of fiberoptics, guided images, microwave, and other technologies to do surgery rather than cutting large sections of tissue.

electrocautery The process of destroying tissue by an electrically heated instrument.

radio frequency ablation (RFA) Uses microwaves to destroy tissue.

Genetic Mapping and Testing

Human Genome Project An international cooperative scientific project to map the 60,000 human genes that make up the human genetic code.

The **Human Genome Project** has provided the driving force behind the explosion of genetic testing possibilities. Geneticists have been able to predict the possibility of genetic disease in a few special circumstances like Huntington's chorea for a long time. Now genetic mapping has given practitioners valuable early information about the possibility of delivering a baby with certain diseases like Down syndrome or Tay-Sachs disease. Genetic mapping can also trace familial history in diseases such as hemophilia. The ability to test for common diseases and disease predisposition and susceptibility for more and more diseases and chronic conditions is becoming available as researchers use the information provided by the Human Genome Project. This will ultimately lead to information about the causes of certain diseases. Even now we have valuable information about the relationship between certain genes and a greater predisposition or susceptibility to disease (www.genome.gov/10002077).

A good example is breast cancer. We now know that women with the genes BRCA1 and/or BRCA2 have a higher probability of getting breast cancer than those women who do not have these genes. Each year more than 192,000 women learn they have breast cancer; 5 percent to 10 percent of those have the hereditary form of breast cancer. According to estimates of lifetime risk, about 13.2 percent (132 out of 1,000 individuals) of women in the general population will develop breast cancer, compared with estimates of 36 percent to 85 percent (360 to 850 out of 1,000) women with an altered BRCA1 or BRCA2 gene. In other words, women with an altered BRCA1 or BRCA2 gene are three to seven times more likely to develop breast cancer than women without alterations in those genes. Women with the genes BRCA1 and/or BRCA2 also have a higher probability of getting ovarian cancer. Lifetime risk estimates of ovarian cancer for women in the general population indicate that 1.7 percent (17 out of 1,000) will get ovarian cancer, compared with 16 percent to 60 percent (160 to 600 out of 1,000) of women with altered BRCA1 or BRCA2 genes (http://www.cancer.gov/about-cancer/causes-prevention/genetics/brca-fact-sheet).

Approximately 500 human genetic diseases can currently be identified by genetic testing. The ability to test for the predisposition to a disease raises important ethical concerns. Insurers would like very much to know who may get a specific disease—it would mean much less risk if the industry could deny insurance to someone on the basis of genetic testing (although the Affordable Care Act prohibits denial on the basis of a preexisting condition). It may be important to people contemplating marriage or business partnerships to know if partners test positive for a specific genetic disease. For the individual, knowing what disease potential he or she has inherited may alter life decisions. In short, genetic testing may result in genetic discrimination.

gene therapy The treatment of disease using normal or altered genes to replace or enhance nonfunctional or missing genes.

Gene Therapy

Gene therapy is a technique for correcting defective genes responsible for disease development. Stem cell therapies, DNA manipulation, genetic alteration through introduction of vector virus, and the repair, replacement, and translocation of genetic material are all covered in this definition. There is ongoing clinical research on both animals and humans.

Gene therapy is an experimental technique that uses genes to treat or prevent disease. In the future, this technique may allow doctors to treat a disorder by inserting a gene into a patient's cells instead of using drugs or surgery. Researchers are testing several approaches to gene therapy, including

- Replacing a mutated gene that causes disease with a healthy copy of the gene
- Inactivating, or "knocking out," a mutated gene that is functioning improperly
- Introducing a new gene into the body to help fight a disease

Although gene therapy is a promising treatment option for a number of diseases (including inherited disorders, some types of cancer, and certain viral infections), the technique remains risky and is still under study to make sure that it will be safe and effective. Gene therapy is currently only being tested for the treatment of diseases that have no other cures (http://ghr.nlm.nih.gov/).

Researchers may use one of several approaches for correcting faulty genes. The most common approach is to insert a normal gene to replace a nonfunctional gene. This is the line of research currently being focused on for type 1 diabetes and Parkinson's disease. Another approach is to swap an abnormal gene for a normal gene through **recombination**. Selective reverse mutation may allow the repair of an abnormal gene, returning it to normal function. The regulation (the degree to which a gene is turned on or off) of a particular gene could be altered. Gene therapy works by using a carrier molecule, called a vector, to deliver the normal gene to the cells. The most common vector is a virus. The virus is introduced to a target organ like the liver, where it injects the new DNA material, theoretically repairing or replacing the defective gene.

recombination The genetic process of new gene combinations that gives rise to offspring that have a combination of genes different from those of either parent.

Cost/Benefit Analysis

The ability to compare patient outcomes with both the specific costs of equipment and training and overall costs of treatment is a vital part of health care economics and policy. The shorthand way of talking about this comparison is a **cost/benefit analysis**. In many countries, a new technology undergoes a formal cost/benefit analysis before being adopted by health care professionals.

cost/benefit analysis The process of comparing the specific costs of a treatment to the benefits obtained by that treatment.

In the United States, the development of new technology is market driven. Companies' ability and interest in developing new products is influenced by FDA requirements and by the availability of insurance coverage for the use of the new technology. However, the lure of that multi-billion dollar market is strong.

On the surface, advanced technology seems like a very expensive way to provide health care. But is it really? In one possible scenario, the new technology can improve individual patient outcomes that make the overall price of the advance to society lower. The second possible scenario is that the use of advanced technology increases the price of care with no improvement of outcomes for patients.

Several examples illustrate these scenarios. The use of laparoscopy surgery has in most cases reduced the overall cost of the procedure by decreasing the hospitalization time from 3 to 7 days down to 1 to 2 days. The cost of the equipment and special training of the physicians and operating room staff is compensated for by the shorter stays. In particular, the overall cost of repair of torn knee cartilage—anterior cruciate ligament repair—using laparoscopic techniques is 75 percent less than the traditional method of repair. However, some of this savings has been possible because the patient now bears a greater burden for postoperative care and rehabilitation. What was once done in the hospital before the patient was discharged is now done at home (Henderson 2014).

In another example, the cost of treating childhood earaches has increased in the last two decades with no significant change in outcomes (Follard, Goodman, and Stano 2012). More consistent application of cost/benefit analysis would help determine if the new technology was really worth it.

Pharmaceuticals

Pharmaceuticals play a key role in modern medicine. The modern drug industry has researched millions of substances looking for new drugs to cure old diseases. Drugs have been used and distributed for thousands of years. Evidence of healing compounds has been found in the archaeological remains of most civilizations. The current pharmaceutical industry began with the discovery of insulin in 1920, the beginning of antibiotics with sulfa and penicillin in the 1930s, and the polio vaccine in the 1950s. It would be hard to imagine life today without the many drugs that save and enhance lives. The other side of the lifesaving coin, however, is people spending their life savings for those very drugs.

Picture of an Industry

prescription drug A drug that must have a health care provider's written order (prescription) to be dispensed.

generic drug A drug sold or dispensed under a name that is not protected by a trademark, usually a chemical name or description (e.g., acetaminophen instead of Tylenol).

over-the-counter (OTC) Drugs and medical devices that may be sold without a written health care provider's order. Aspirin and crutches are examples.

Three major types of drugs produced can broadly categorize the pharmaceutical industry: prescription, generic, and over-the-counter (OTC). **Prescription drugs** are those available when a physician prescribes them for a patient and a pharmacist fills the prescription. Because the manufacturer of the drug holds a patent on the drug that gives the manufacturer the sole right to produce that drug, the sale of prescription drugs is enormously profitable. In fact, manufacturers rely on their so-called blockbuster drugs for as much as 45 percent of their company profits.

Generic drugs are those drugs that no longer have patent protection; therefore, any company can manufacture essentially the same drug under its company name. Generics are generally much cheaper than a brand-name alternative. **Over-the-counter (OTC)** medications are those that consumers can buy for themselves without a prescription, and they include both brand-name and generic equivalents. Examples are Tagamet (cimetidine), Benadryl, cortisone topical ointment, and Motrin. Many prescription drugs are also available in an OTC form.

To bring a prescription drug to market, three major functions occur in a pharmaceutical company: research and development (R&D), production, and sales and marketing. In the R&D function, scientists work to develop new drugs (the complete process is described later in the chapter). Most of these researchers are highly trained, holding PhDs or MDs, and companies invest in additional training so that their researchers stay current in their fields. In 2014, companies spent an estimated $51.2 billion on R&D, reinvesting 17.9 percent of sales revenue into this critical activity (Pharmaceutical Research and Manufacturers of America 2015). As the R&D process identifies candidates for potential drugs, the production function begins to analyze whether the drug can be produced in sufficient quantity and quality to be profitable. Many of the personnel involved in this function have engineering backgrounds. The sales and marketing function designs a strategy to get the word out about the drug. Specific strategies are discussed later in the chapter. Companies recruit sales representatives with bachelor's degrees in the sciences and then extensively train them about the company's products.

According to data from the National Center for Health Statistics, 75 percent of office visits involved drug therapy, with 2.6 million drugs ordered or provided. The three most commonly prescribed classes of drugs are analgesics, antihyperlipidemic agents, and antidepressants. In the past 30 days, 48 percent of people have used at least one prescription drug, 21 percent use three or more, and 10 percent use five or more (National Center for Health Statistics 2015). This level of consumption translates into an industry that is extremely profitable. Table 11.2 describes the world's largest pharmaceutical companies; non–U.S. companies are included because this is truly a global industry.

Table 11.2 | *Largest Pharmaceutical Companies, 2014*

Company (Country)	Sales[i]	R&D Spending	Profits	Employees
Johnson & Johnson (USA)	$74.3	$8.5	$16.3	126.5
Pfizer (USA)	49.4	7.2	9.1	78
GlaxoSmithKline (UK)	23.0 (L)	3.5 (L)	3.6 (L)	97.9
Roche Group (SF)	47.5 (CHF)	8.9 (CHF)	53 (CHF)	88.5
Sanofi-Aventis (FR)	33.8€	4.8€	4.4€	113.5
AstraZeneca (UK)	26.1	5.3	6.9	57.5
Abbott Labs (USA)	20.2	1.4	2.3	72
Merck (USA)	42.2	7.2	11.9	70
Abbvie (IR)	19.96	3.3	1.8	26
Bristol-Myers Squibb (USA)	15.9	4.5	2.0	28
Eli Lilly (USA)	19.6	4.73	2.39	39.1

Source: Company reports
Note: Sales, R&D, and Profits in $billions, except where foreign currency is indicated; Employees in 1,000s. SF Switzerland (CHF average 2014 rate at $0.95); FR France (euro average 2014 rate at $1.32); IR Ireland; UK United Kingdom (pounds sterling average 2014 rate at $1.60).

All these companies are publicly traded and must file quarterly reports, known as 10-ks, with the Securities and Exchange Commission. The reports are available online and provide significant disclosure of the company's financials.

Industry Regulation

The pharmaceutical industry is one of the most heavily regulated industries in the United States. The Food and Drug Act of 1906 was passed in response to public outcry against dangerous food additives and drugs. The act did not require testing for safety, only that drugs and food additions be labeled with their major ingredient. In 1938, the federal Food, Drug and Cosmetic Act began requiring testing for safety. The act left the responsibility for the testing to the drug companies, requiring only reporting of testing. It was not until 1959 and the Kefauver Senate hearings on the questionable practices of drug companies that further legislation was introduced.

The thalidomide tragedy occurred shortly after these hearings. Thalidomide was a tranquilizer used in early pregnancy to control nausea and vomiting. It was widely used in Europe prior to its introduction to the United States. Soon there were reports of severe birth defects. The drug was available for experimental use in the United States. The FDA withdrew approval for the drug but not before some children were born with these defects.

In response to the tragedy, in 1962 Congress passed amendments to the 1938 Act to give much more control to the FDA over the introduction of new products. The new powers required more extensive testing of new drugs and controlled the premarket distribution of new drugs more tightly. The process for new drug distribution has become a multistage process that takes a number of years and is quite expensive. In addition, the FDA also has the authority to regulate drug advertising.

Getting a New Drug to Market

The road from a molecule discovered in a plant or animal to a marketable drug is a long one. Table 11.3 presents the complete process, described in detail next.

Table 11.3	*The Drug Development Process*	
Stage of Development	**No. Compounds**	**Years**
Drug discovery	Millions	5
Preclinical	250	1.5
Clinical trials		
Phase I	1–5	2–10
Phase II		total for
Phase III		trials
FDA review	1 drug approved	2
Large-scale manufacturing		2
Phase IV		

Through the new tool of **gene sequencing**, scientists can examine millions of compounds in a year to screen for good ideas or drug leads. Out of these come perhaps 10,000 that are tested; 1,000 of these show bioactivity; of these maybe 100 are worth investigating; from there, 10 go to clinical trials; maybe then 1 of those millions of compounds ends up as a drug on the shelf.

Once a drug company decides a new drug has potential, it must file an **investigational new drug (IND) application** with the FDA to begin clinical tests on human subjects. The three phases of clinical tests are designed to answer three primary questions:

1. Is the new drug safe?
2. Does it work?
3. Is it better than the standard treatment already in place?

Scientists who want to test drugs on people to answer these questions must follow strict rules to make sure that the drug is as safe as possible. The National Institutes of Health (NIH) website provides the information that volunteers must receive before they are selected for a **clinical trial** (www.nih.gov). The clinical trial is designed and then must be approved by an **Institutional Review Board (IRB)**. These boards review all human experimentation. The volunteers must give informed consent and sign a form that says they understand the risks and benefits of the study.

To this point, the process has taken several years. The three-phase testing process required by the FDA can now begin and will take several more years to complete. Currently hundreds of drugs are in process.

Phase I tests the drug to figure out what happens to the drug in the body. How is the drug absorbed, metabolized, and excreted? Blood, urine, and timing tests are done on the volunteers; there may be as few as a dozen or as many as 100. This phase takes several months. If there are no serious adverse effects, then after review, the next phase begins.

Phase II studies whether the drug produces the desired effect. For example, does it stop the pain of a migraine or reduce the size of a tumor? This phase may take several years and involves several hundred patients. Patients are carefully monitored for both the desired effect and side effects such as nausea, headaches, or heart irregularities.

Tests in Phase II and III are often conducted in **blind random trials**. The volunteers do not know whether they are receiving the drug, a placebo, or the standard treatment. Neither does the physician who examines the volunteers. This type of trial prevents preconceptions from biasing the results.

Phase III typically lasts several years and involves thousands of patients in different parts of the country. The safety and effectiveness of the drug compared to both the standard treatment and placebos are carefully analyzed and studied. Occasionally a clinical trial is halted and the trial unblinded, if the results indicate either the drug could save lives or there are serious complications.

If all phases go well, the drug company submits a **New Drug Application (NDA)** to the FDA for approval to market the drug. During Phase IV, the

gene sequencing
The process of determining the individual arrangement of nucleotides that compose a given gene. Used extensively in drug research.

investigational new drug (IND) application
The notice to the FDA (Food and Drug Administration) that a company intends to begin clinical tests on humans.

clinical trial The process of testing a new drug, treatment, or medical device on humans in a controlled manner.

Institutional Review Board (IRB) The group of people appointed by the government or a university to oversee any research on animals or humans.

blind random trials A clinical trial method in which no one knows which drugs the participants are receiving until the trial is finished.

New Drug Application (NDA)
The formal request to the FDA to be allowed to market a new drug.

From Fish to Pharmacies: A Story of Drug Development

A diet rich in calcium is supposed to keep your bones strong and prevent osteoporosis, a disease characterized by bone mass deterioration. Most of the 2 million Americans affected by the disease are women. The disease may be responsible for 5 million fractures of the hip, wrist, and spine in people over 50 and may cause 50,000 deaths. According to the National Osteoporosis Foundation, that costs $13.8 billion a year.

The thyroid gland secretes a hormone called calcitonin that regulates calcium and decreases bone loss. As it turns out salmon make calcitonin too, but it's 30 times more potent than what humans make. Better yet, you can make synthetic salmon calcitonin in a lab, which is a simpler and cheaper way to make a lot of the product than using real fish. To find out if the salmon calcitonin would make a good drug to fight osteoporosis, drug developers followed the FDA approval process.

The FDA approved the first drug based on salmon calcitonin in an injectable. Since then, two more drugs, one injectable and one administered through a nasal spray, were approved. An oral version of salmon calcitonin is in clinical trials now. Salmon calcitonin is approved only for postmenopausal women who cannot tolerate estrogen, or for whom estrogen is not an option.

Source: Adapted from http://www.fda.gov/Drugs/DevelopmentApprovalProcess/HowDrugsareDevelopedandApproved/default.htm.

FDA continues to monitor the drug. After the drug is on the market, if any problems arise, the manufacturer is required to file adverse incident reports with the FDA. The responsibility of physicians and health care facilities to report is voluntary. The FDA received 1.18 million reports in 2013 (http://www.fda.gov/Drugs/GuidanceComplianceRegulatoryInformation/Surveillance/AdverseDrugEffects/; http://www.fda.gov/Safety/MedWatch/default.htm).

The FDA can recall a drug when a clear threat to patient safety exists. For example, the anticholesterol drug Baycol was recalled after several patients died from complications caused by the drug. A complete list of withdrawals and recalls is available from the FDA (http://www.fda.gov/safety/recalls/default.htm).

Sales and Marketing Efforts

After a drug is approved for market, the drug company must get it into the patients' hands. Typically there are three major ways to market a new drug in the United States. Two strategies target the physicians who prescribe the drug, and one targets patients directly.

The first way to market a new drug is by medical journal and conference reporting on the new drug. This approach is targeted to the physicians who specialize in the disease for which the drug is under investigation. *The New England Journal of Medicine* and *Lancet* (in Great Britain) are examples of juried publications that report on drug research. Reports of the benefits of the drugs in medical journals may begin while the drug is in Phase III testing.

The second major tool is personal selling by drug representatives of pharmaceutical companies. Drug representatives call on physicians to solicit their use of the drug (see this chapter's career profile for more information). This may be accompanied by free samples of the drugs for patients and literature and promotional material advertising the drug. Many offices never purchase pens or note pads because so many are given away by the drug representatives. Members of the Pharmaceutical Research and Manufacturers of America, an industry trade group, have adopted a voluntary code that governs interactions with health care professionals. Giveaway items that bear a company or product name are allowed if the items "entail a benefit to patients" and "are primarily associated with the health care professional's practice." Although the code allows members to provide informational presentations to health care professionals, the code prohibits entertainment/recreational events, takeout meals, and the inclusion of spouses or guests. Because these codes are voluntary, there is no enforcement mechanism if a member violates the code.

The third way is to reach patients directly by paid advertising. The United States is the only country that allows advertising of prescription drugs. Advertising was confined to the professional journals but is now common in popular magazines like *Newsweek* and *People*. A comprehensive advertising campaign includes television and the Web as well as print ads.

Despite the fact that various universities and government agencies have studied the question, it is unclear whether drug advertising drives up the cost of pharmaceuticals. Only a handful of the most popular drugs are advertised in the popular media, but those have advertising budgets in the millions. Claritin, Lipitor, and Viagra are examples of drugs advertised in popular print and television media. Generic drugs are not advertised. According to surveys of physicians, patients often now ask for drugs by brand name. These drugs are usually more expensive than the lesser-known drugs of the same family.

The FDA regulates direct-to-consumer advertisements of prescription drugs; in addition, the Federal Trade Commission (FTC) regulates truth in advertising generally. The FDA requires that direct-to-consumer advertising be accurate and not misleading, make claims only if supported by substantial evidence, reflect a balance of risks and benefits, and be consistent with FDA-approved labeling (PhRMA 2009).

The Cost of Prescription Drugs

The economic success of pharmaceutical companies and the high cost of prescription drugs have caused considerable media attention to be focused on the industry. To save money, 15 percent of adults asked for a lower-cost prescription, 8 percent did not take the medicine as prescribed, 4 percent used alternative therapies, and almost 2 percent bought prescription drugs from another country (Cohen and Villarroel 2015). Cost-containment strategies are being used in all countries to try to slow down the upward trend in drug costs. The strategies include switching to generic drugs, legislation, more cost/benefit analysis, and awareness by practitioners of costs.

The switch to generic drugs instead of brand names is one major way to control costs. Eighty-six percent of prescriptions are filled with a generic option. The

Affordable Care Act's emphasis on prevention has made some significant improvements. More than half of all prescriptions cost less than $5, with 23 percent available at no out-of-pocket expense (IMS 2014). Common preventive medicine and oral contraceptives are the largest "free" categories. The estimated saving for contraceptives in 2013 was $483 million. This is balanced against high-cost specialty medicines and those in the doughnut hole of Medicare D; 30 percent of out-of-pocket costs came from just 2.3 percent of prescriptions. Over a third of prescription spending is on just five therapies: oncology, antidiabetes, mental health, respiratory agents, and pain.

Another strategy is for independent research facilities to do serious cost/benefit analysis by comparing drugs in the same family to determine if the more you pay, the more you get. Most of these studies have shown that price is not the quality determinant. In one Australian study, the least-expensive drug showed no significant difference in patient outcomes among three drugs in the same family for gastric reflux and esophageal reflux. Changing to the least-expensive drug that gives a good outcome can save millions of dollars a year.

Finally, health practitioners need to be aware of pricing when prescribing. One NIH study demonstrates that physicians rarely ask the patients if they can afford the drug they are prescribing; consequently, patients often do not fill the prescription because they cannot pay for it. For instance, the top-selling drug for gastric reflux, pantoprazole, may cost $541 for a month's supply, whereas a generic pump inhibitor may only cost $100 per month. For a person on a fixed budget, this is the difference between eating or paying the rent and buying the drug. If the physician or nurse practitioner is not sensitive to drug pricing, the patient may not get needed medication. As noted in Chapter 4 , changes to Medicare Part D have increased the access of older Americans to prescription medications, just as the Affordable Care Act has increased the access of people who previously lacked insurance.

Social and Ethical Questions

The high cost of drug therapy not only spurs efforts to contain costs, but also raises the issue of whether industry profits are excessive. The industry has argued that patent protection and profitability are the return firms receive for the investment they made in the research and production process. As you have read earlier in this chapter, the process to bring a new prescription drug to market is both long and costly. The industry argues that without patent protection (essentially a short-term monopoly), they would be unable to afford the cost and risks associated with the process. The industry also argues that the price they charge is a way to recover those costs, as well as the legal and financial risks once a drug is available to the market. As many primary patents expire, the drug companies are just now experiencing the pressures of competition. Ongoing mergers in the pharmaceutical industry reflect the search for better profitability. Consumers, the media, and politicians question pricing policies and may not accept the industry's arguments.

There is an urgent need for the increased research and development of new drugs. The emergence of worldwide epidemics such as HIV/AIDS,

Ebola, avian or bird flu, and West Nile disease requires new vaccines or new antibiotics. The rise in numbers of patients with antibiotic-resistant tuberculosis (TB) and staphylococcus infections indicates pharmaceutical emergencies. These conditions have a high mortality rate and are not responding to traditional drug therapy. How should drug companies be reimbursed for the research and development of vaccines and drugs to combat these and new emerging epidemics?

The controversy over HIV/AIDS drugs is only the first in a long line of social and ethical questions about drug therapy. Should millions die because the drugs to treat AIDS are too expensive for most countries, let alone individuals, to afford? The cost for a year of AIDS drugs in the United States is over $40,000, many times over the average annual income worldwide. More than 1 million people in the United States and 40 million worldwide have AIDS. Most of the new cases are in developing nations and minority populations in the developed countries (http://www.niaid.nih.gov/about/organization/daids/).

Many advocate that patents on certain drugs, such as those for AIDS, malaria, and TB, should be canceled. The research should be available to everyone, following the model of the Human Genome Project. The pricing of drugs that only have a very limited market for distribution for people with rare diseases is another area of concern. The price of the generation of drugs that brings together genetic research and targeted cell response will probably remain high. These and many more questions are issues for those making social policy around the world.

Career Profile: Pharmaceuticals Sales Representative

One of the primary ways that pharmaceutical companies get the word out about their products is through their sales reps. If you have good organizational and people skills and a knowledge of the medical field, then a career as a pharmaceuticals sales representative might be for you.

On a day-to-day basis reps work with health care professionals such as physicians and office staff. They spend time calling on their customers, both on the phone and in person, to build a relationship so they can meet the needs of the health care professional and the patient. They use their selling skills to convince the physician to prescribe the drugs made by the company they represent. They distribute samples and product literature. And they keep good records of their activities.

Although there are occasionally jobs that require an associate's degree in nursing or related field, most entry-level jobs require a bachelor's or higher degree. It helps to have had sales experience. You should be able to work independently, and travel is required. Jobs are available in locations across the country. In 2015 entry-level positions earned $50,000. Senior representatives with specialized knowledge and experience can earn $130,000. This career has a good upward career ladder with many opportunities for career advancement and geographic locations.

Summary

Medical technology is those therapeutic and diagnostic devices used by health professionals to prevent, treat, and diagnose illness and assist patients medically. Pharmaceuticals are the research, production, marketing, and dispensing of agents (drugs, genes, molecules, etc.) that are bioactive in the human body for therapeutic purposes. Medical technology and pharmaceuticals have had a huge impact on modern health care, both in improving individual patient outcomes and in the increase in spending on health care.

New medical technologies include medical devices such as pacemakers, insulin pumps, new imaging techniques, computer-assisted imaging, new drugs, and genetic mapping and testing. New types of pharmaceuticals will use DNA manipulation and stem cell research. Pharmaceuticals can now target individual receptors and cells.

The pharmaceutical industry is a global industry with a huge financial impact. Companies research millions of possibilities to arrive at one marketable drug. A new drug gets to market through a three-phase testing and research process that may take 10 to 12 years. Ethical issues include the cost of prescription drugs and new medical technologies as well as the decision to research and develop drugs for certain diseases and not for others.

Questions for Review

1. Define the terms and give examples of medical technology and pharmaceuticals.
2. Describe four new medical technologies.
3. What is the difference between prescription, generic, and over-the-counter (OTC) drugs?
4. Describe two ways pharmaceuticals are marketed.
5. Using a flowchart, explain how a new drug gets to market.

Questions for Discussion

1. What is the impact of medical technology and pharmaceuticals on modern health care? Use comparisons in your answer.
2. How is the pharmaceutical industry regulated? Do you believe that this process safeguards the public's health?
3. Do some cost research of your own. Pick a drug, and compare the cost of at least two suppliers. What accounts for the differences?
4. Should patents be available on drugs that can save people's lives?
5. Who should decide which medical technologies and which pharmaceuticals are developed?
6. Should stem cell research for diseases like Parkinson's be available to scientists all over the world like the Human Genome Project—why/why not?

Chapter References

Bryan, J. 1996. *The history of health and medicine: Advances that have changed the world.* Austin, TX: Raintree Steck-Vaughn.

Centers for Disease Control and Prevention (www.cdc.gov).

CDC, Health Statistics. 2009. *Chartbook. Health, United States. Special feature: Medical technology.* Atlanta, GA: Author.

Cohen, R., and M. Villarroel. 2015. *Strategies used by adults to reduce their prescription drug costs: United States, 2013.* NCHS Data Brief, 184. January. Available at http://www.cdc.gov/nchs/data/databriefs/db184.pdf.

http://www.fda.gov/Drugs/DevelopmentApprovalProcess/default.htm.

http://www.fda.gov/Drugs/DevelopmentApprovalProcess/HowDrugsareDevelopedandApproved/default.htm.

http://www.fda.gov/Drugs/GuidanceComplianceRegulatoryInformation/Surveillance/AdverseDrugEffects/.

http://www.fda.gov/Safety/MedWatch/default.htm.

http://www.fda.gov/safety/recalls/default.htm.

Follard, S., A. Goodman, and M. Stano. 2012. *The economics of health and health care.* 7th ed. Upper Saddle River, NJ: Prentice Hall.

Genetics Home Reference (http://ghr.nlm.nih.gov/).

www.genome.gov/10002077.

Henderson, J. 2014. *Health economics and policy.* 6th ed. Stamford, CT: Cengage Learning.

IMS Institute. 2014. *Medicine use and shifting costs of healthcare: A review of the use of medicines in the United States in 2013.* April. Available at http://www.imshealth.com/deployedfiles/imshealth/Global/Content/Corporate/IMS%20Health%20Institute/Reports/Secure/IIHI_US_Use_of_Meds_for_2013.pdf.

National Cancer Institute (http://www.cancer.gov/about-cancer/causes-prevention/genetics/brca-fact-sheet).

National Center for Health Statistics. 2015. *Health, United States, 2014.* Hyattsville, MD: Table 85.

National Institute of Allergy and Infectious Disease, National Institutes of Health, Division of Acquired Immunodeficiency Syndrome (www.niaid.nih.gov/daids/).

National Institutes of Health (www.nih.gov).

National Institutes of Health, Clinical Center, Diagnostic Radiology Department (www.cc.nih.gov/drd/rfa/background.html).

National Institutes of Health, Stem Cell Information (http://stemcells.nih.gov/info/basics/).

http://www.ncbi.nlm.nih.gov/pmc/articles/PMC3549771/.

Pharmaceutical Research and Manufacturers of America (PhRMA). 2015. *Biopharmaceutical industry profile 2010.* Available at http://www.phrma.org/sites/default/files/pdf/2015_phrma_profile.pdf.

_____. 2009. *PhRMA guiding principles: Direct to consumer advertisements about prescription medicines.* Available at http://phrma.org/sites/default/files/pdf/phrmaguidingprinciplesdec08final.pdf.

U.S. Census Bureau. 2013. *Annual survey of manufactures. NAICS 3391.*

For Additional Information

Danis, M., C. Clancy, and L. Churchill. 2003. *Ethical dimensions of health policy.* New York: Oxford University Press.

Li, J. 2014. *Blockbuster drugs: The rise and decline of the pharmaceutical industry.* New York: Oxford University Press.

Werth, B. 2014. *The antidote: Inside the world of new pharma.* New York: Simon & Schuster.

12

Health Care Research and Prevention

Learning Objectives

After reading this chapter, you should be able to:

1. Identify the three major goals of health research.
2. Describe the process of obtaining a research grant from NIH.
3. Explain the role of the government in prevention.
4. Identify the top 10 causes of death in the United States.
5. Research a health care topic using Web resources.
6. Discuss the *Healthy People 2020* goals.

Fighting the Flu

One of the types of prevention most of us have practiced is the annual flu shot. This is one of the most common preventive pharmaceuticals in the world. Each year, millions of people line up to be vaccinated for the flu. In 2009, 126 million people were vaccinated against the new H1N1 influenza (www.flu.gov).

The flu or influenza is viral infection caused by a specific virus. The Centers for Disease Control and Prevention (CDC) estimates that 10 to 20 percent of Americans come down with the flu during each flu season, which typically lasts from the beginning of November through March. Children are two to three times more likely than adults to contract the disease and are often the means by which the disease is spread to both other children and adults. The CDC further estimates that 100,000 people are hospitalized and 36,000 people die annually from the flu and its complications. Table 12.1 lists the major pandemics.

The Influenza Virus

The influenza virus is wound with eight segments of single-strand RNA inside, which is responsible for copying the virus. When viewed under an electron microscope, the most striking feature of the virus is a layer of spikes projecting from its surface. There are two different types of spikes: one is the protein hemagglutinin HA(H), which allows the virus to stick to a cell and begin infection; the other is a protein called neuraminidase NA(N), which enables newly formed viruses to leave the host cell and infect new cells. These spikes allow the virus to shed or drop from the body of the infected person or animal and easily infect other people or animals.

Depending on their protein composition, influenza viruses are classified as type A, B, or C. Found in many kinds of animals, including chickens, ducks, pigs, whales, and humans, type A is not only the most common flu virus, but also the most deadly of the three types. Type A was responsible for the global human pandemics of 1918, 1957, 1968, and 2009/2010, which killed millions of people. The avian, or bird, flu is a type A virus; it kills millions of wild migratory and domestic chickens and ducks, and when it mutates, it causes worldwide human flu epidemics. The year 2015 saw a huge outbreak in the United States, affecting over 48 million birds in 15 states (http://www.aphis.usda.gov/wps/portal/aphis/ourfocus/animalhealth/sa_animal_disease_information/sa_avian_health/ct_avian_influenza_disease).

Type A viruses are divided into subtypes depending on the host (chicken, duck, etc.), the place first found, a laboratory identification number, the year of discovery, the place of origin, and, in parentheses, the surface spikes; the Hong Kong flu of 1997 is thus known as A/Chicken/Hong Kong/G9/97 (H9N2). This scientific notation allows the scientific community to communicate rapidly about which flu is being researched and to identify new strains quickly. This ability to track new viruses is important because the type A virus periodically undergoes sudden and dramatic changes that create new subtypes. Because the change is so sudden, people have no immunity to the new subtypes. Severe epidemics are the result, as in 1918, 1957, 1968, and 2009/2010.

The H1N1 pandemic of 2009 was a type A virus. In April 2009, human infection with a new strain of H1N1 influenza was confirmed in Mexico. Within weeks, human infections spread to the United States, and cases began occurring in other regions around the world. In the United States, the CDC estimated there were 57 million cases of H1N1 flu between April 2009 and January 2010, with 275,000 people hospitalized and 11,600 deaths in that period. 2014 was a particularly severe season with the highest number of hospitalizations, particularly in the 65+ age group, since flu surveillance began.

The type B virus causes epidemics, but the disease it produces is milder than those caused by type A. A new vaccine must be developed each year because B viruses have gradual and continuous changes, called antigenic drift. Although these changes are not dramatic, they make the new virus unrecognizable to the human immune system. Type C virus has been found in humans, pigs, and dogs (dog flu). This virus causes a mild respiratory infection but does not spark epidemics.

The flu virus has been in the wild aquatic bird population for millions of years and normally does not harm the birds. However, when the virus mutates, it can quickly jump from wild birds to the domestic duck and chicken population. From there, the next step is for the virus to jump species and infect a new host, usually the pig. This is because pigs, ducks, and chickens are frequently found together on domestic farms around the world. Humans, chickens, ducks, and pigs may all carry any one of the three flu viruses. If the pig gets the human and the avian virus together, a genetic exchange takes place, and a new virus is formed. This resulting form of the virus may then spread from the pigs to humans and then from humans to humans. In 1997, scientists found the first instance of the avian flu skipping the pig stage and going straight to humans. The severity of the flu is determined by the ability of the virus to be spread from human to human.

The symptoms of the flu don't actually begin until about 4 days after a person has been exposed and infected. During this period and for the first 3 to 4 days after the first symptoms, the person is contagious. Because the person doesn't realize he or she is sick, it is easy to see why the flu spreads so quickly in schools and workplaces. The symptoms usually start quickly with a fever, body aches, chills, dry cough, headache, sore throat, and stuffy nose. The fever is the highest for the first 3 days. The respiratory symptoms may last several weeks, depending on the type of virus. The stomach flu is not influenza. The diagnosis is usually made on the basis of the symptoms and the known extent of the epidemic. Laboratory tests are not often used for routine diagnosis, but they can be used early in the epidemic to determine which type of virus is responsible for the epidemic.

The best way to prevent the flu is to get a flu shot 6 to 8 weeks before the season starts. The yearly flu vaccine is made up of the killed A and B type viruses the scientists feel will most likely be in circulation that year. This determination is made about 9 months before the North American flu season begins in November. The better the tracking of the flu virus, the better the vaccines are against it.

How are the viruses selected to make flu vaccine? The viruses used in making seasonal flu vaccines are chosen each year based on information collected over the previous year about which influenza viruses are spreading and what vaccine viruses would offer the best protection against circulating viruses. Viruses gathered by 130 national influenza centers in

101 countries as well as information on disease trends are further analyzed by the four World Health Organization (WHO) Collaborating Centers for Reference and Research on Influenza located in Atlanta, United States (CDC); London, United Kingdom (National Institute for Medical Research); Melbourne, Australia (Victoria Infectious Diseases Reference Laboratory); and Tokyo, Japan (National Institute for Infectious Diseases). The seasonal flu vaccine is usually a trivalent vaccine (a three-component vaccine), with each component selected to protect against one of the three groups of influenza viruses circulating most commonly in humans.

In a trivalent vaccine, the three vaccine viruses are chosen to maximize the likelihood that the main circulating viruses during the upcoming flu season will be well covered by the vaccine. The WHO recommends specific vaccine viruses for vaccine production, but then each individual country makes its own decision for licensing of vaccines in its country. In the United States, the U.S. Food and Drug Administration (FDA) determines what viruses will be used in U.S.–licensed vaccines. For instance in 2016 the mix was made to protect against the following three viruses:

- A/California/7/2009 (H1N1)pdm09-like virus
- A/Switzerland/9715293/2013 (H3N2)-like virus
- B/Phuket/3073/2013-like virus (This is a B/Yamagata lineage virus.)

Some of the 2015–2016 flu vaccine was quad-rivalent vaccine and also protects against an additional B virus (B/Brisbane/60/2008-like virus). This is a B/Victoria lineage virus.

Even though you have been vaccinated, you may still get the flu; the symptoms are milder in those who have had the shot.

Since 2004, there have been periodic shortages of the vaccine, particularly in 2009 for the H1N1 flu vaccine. However, the production of flu vaccine has improved; as many as 174 million doses will be manufactured for U.S. consumption for the 2016 season. Other methods for prevention have been recommended. In 2003, the FDA approved a live virus nasal spray vaccine called FluMist, which can be used for healthy people between the ages of 5 and 49. There are also antiviral medicines available by prescription, such as Tamiflu (oseltamivir), Flumadine (rimantadine), and Symmetrel (amantadine), that will help prevent flu infection if you take them for at least 2 weeks during the outbreak. Rimantadine and amantadine can be used in persons 1 year or older, but oseltamivir is for adults and teenagers 13 years and older. There have been reports of drug resistance to the H1N1 virus.

New research suggests that increased dietary use of whole grains and exercise helps in preventing the flu. Nevertheless, the treatment for the flu has not changed much in the last 50 years. Doctors recommend bed rest, fluids, and acetaminophen for fever and body aches. But prevention is actually the best medicine.

Source: http:www.flu.gov; http://www.cdc.gov/flu/weekly/summary.htm; http://www.cdc.gov/flu/about/season/flu-season-2015-2016.htm

Introduction

Throughout this text, you have learned that the function of the health care industry is to diagnose and treat illness. As indicated in the chapter profile, research and tracking of disease play an important role in being able to control and cure illness. In this chapter, the research side of health care is presented. And because it is better if people don't get sick to begin with, the chapter looks at prevention as an increasingly central health care strategy.

Table 12.1	*Influenza Timeline*
	Appearance of a New Influenza Strain in the Human Population

antigenic drift
Describes the gradual and continuous changes in the genetic makeup of some viruses such as the type B flu virus.

1918   Pandemic
"Spanish flu" H1N1

> The most devastating flu pandemic in recent history, killing more than 500,000 people in the United States and 20 million to 50 million people worldwide.

1957–58 Pandemic
"Asian flu" H2N2

> First identified in China, this virus caused roughly 70,000 deaths in the United States during the 1957–58 season. Because this strain has not circulated in humans since 1968, no one younger than 30 years old has immunity to this strain.

1968–69 Pandemic
"Hong Kong flu" H3N2

> First detected in Hong Kong, this virus caused roughly 34,000 deaths in the United States during the 1968–69 season. H3N2 viruses still circulate today.

1977   Appearance of a new influenza strain in humans
"Russian flu" H1N1

> Isolated in northern China, this virus was similar to the virus that spread before 1957. For this reason, individuals born before 1957 were generally protected; children and young adults born after that year, however, were not because they had no prior immunity.

1997   Appearance of a new influenza strain in humans
H5N1

> The first time an influenza virus was found to be transmitted directly from birds to people, with infections linked to exposure to poultry markets. Eighteen people in Hong Kong were hospitalized, six of whom died.

H9N2

> Caused illness in two children in Hong Kong, with poultry the probable source.

2002   Appearance of a new influenza strain in humans
H7N2

> Evidence of infection is found in one person in Virginia following a poultry outbreak.

(continued)

Table 12.1	*Influenza Timeline (continued)*

2003 H5N1	**Appearance of a new influenza strain in humans**
	Caused two Hong Kong family members to be hospitalized after a visit to China, killing one of them, a 33-year-old man. (A third family member died while in China of an undiagnosed respiratory illness.)
H7N7	Eighty-nine people in the Netherlands, most of whom were poultry workers, became ill with eye infections or flu-like symptoms. A veterinarian who visited one of the affected poultry farms died.
H7N2	Caused a person to be hospitalized in New York.
H9N2	Caused illness in one child in Hong Kong.
2004 H5N1	**Appearance of a new influenza strain in humans**
	Caused illness in 47 people in Thailand and Vietnam, 34 of whom died. Researchers are especially concerned because this flu strain, which is quite deadly, is becoming endemic in Asia.
H7N3	Is reported for the first time in humans. The strain caused illness in two poultry workers in Canada.
H10N7	Is reported for the first time in humans. It caused illness in two infants in Egypt. One child's father is a poultry merchant.
2005 H5N1	The first case of human infection with H5N1 arises in Cambodia in February. By May, WHO reports four Cambodian cases, all fatal. Indonesia reports its first case, which is fatal, in July. Over the next 3 months, seven cases of laboratory-confirmed H5N1 infection in Indonesia, and four deaths, occur.
	On December 30, WHO reports a cumulative total of 142 laboratory-confirmed cases of H5N1 infection worldwide, all in Asia, with 74 deaths. Asian countries in which human infection with H5N1 has been detected: Thailand, Vietnam, Cambodia, Indonesia, and China.
2006 H5N1	In early January, two human cases of H5N1 infection, both fatal, are reported in rural areas of Eastern Turkey, while cases in China continue to spread. As of January 25, China reports a total of 10 cases, with 7 deaths. On January 30, Iraq reports its first case of human H5N1 infection, which was fatal, to WHO.
	In March, WHO confirmed seven cases of human H5N1 infection, and five deaths, in Azerbaijan. In April, WHO confirmed four cases of human H5N1 infection, and two fatalities, in Egypt.

Table 12.1	*(continued)*

In May, WHO confirmed a case of human H5N1 infection in the African nation of Djibouti. This was the first confirmed case in sub-Saharan Africa. Throughout 2006, 115 human cases of H5N1 infection occur, with 79 deaths.

2007

H5N1

In early January, two human cases of H5N1 are confirmed in Indonesia. By the end of 2007, 88 confirmed cases occur in Indonesia, Cambodia, China, Lao People's Democratic Republic, Myanmar, Nigeria, Pakistan, and Vietnam, with 59 deaths.

H7N7

In May, four cases of H7N7 avian influenza were confirmed in the United Kingdom among individuals exposed to infected poultry.

2008

H5N1

On May 28, Bangladesh reports its first case of human H5N1 infection to WHO. By the end of the year, 40 cases are confirmed in Bangladesh, Cambodia, China, Egypt, Indonesia, and Vietnam.

2009

H5N1

On January 7, Indonesia confirmed a new case of human infection with H5N1 influenza. Since that time, new cases have been identified in Egypt, China, Indonesia, and Vietnam.

H1N1

In April, human infection with a new strain of H1N1 influenza is confirmed in Mexico. Within weeks, human infections spread to the United States, and cases begin occurring in other regions around the world.

2014–15

Highest recorded number of hospitalizations since record keeping began.

2015

Avian flu infected over 50 million birds in the United States.

Source: http://www3.niaid.nih.gov/topics/Flu/Research/Pandemic/TimelineHuman Pandemics.htm; http://www.aphis.usda.gov/wps/portal/aphis/ourfocus/animal health/sa_animal_disease_information/sa_avian_health/ct_avian_influenza_disease; http://www.cdc.gov/flu/weekly/summary.htm

Health Care Research: A Pound of Cure

To know what to do to prevent a condition or disease, a person must first know what are the causes, or **predispositions**. That is the job of health care research. Researchers not only find the cures for bacterial diseases like strep throat or bacterial meningitis, but they also learn how to control symptoms and prevent the condition in the first place.

predisposition
In medicine, a susceptibility to a disease or condition because of hereditary or other factors.

Medical research is conducted in several settings in the United States. Faculty at the major research universities, such as the University of Washington, Harvard University, and the University of Maryland, is one group who conducts research. The research can be government sponsored or supported by funds from private industry or from not-for-profit organizations. Research is also conducted by scientists at the National Institutes of Health (NIH) laboratories, the CDC laboratories, and other research-based public institutions. As you saw in Chapter 11, private industry also conducts research.

Types of Research

curative research
Research whose major aim is to find a cure for a specific disease.

Research can be classified by its goal. Generally, the three goals are cure, control, and prevention. **Curative research** is designed to eliminate a disease altogether. This type of research may be done through either physical treatments or pharmaceuticals. Physical treatments include various surgical procedures, such as those that either eliminate tumors or correct abnormalities. Correction of congenital heart abnormalities is an ongoing type of curative surgical research. The use of laser robotic surgery for organ removal such as a hysterectomy is another example of current surgical research.

Curative research can focus on the use of pharmaceuticals such as antibiotics that eliminate disease. Antibiotics are very good at eliminating bacterial disease and one of the few areas where medication alone can cure a disease. A current subject of curative pharmaceutical research is macular degeneration, a vision problem that causes loss of sight in the center of the visual field through destruction of the retina. There are two types of macular degeneration, dry and wet. Dry is the most common form; as of yet there is no cure, only minimal control by vitamins and minerals. Several drugs, including Avastin, Lucentis, Macugen, Eylea, iSONEP, and MC-1101, are in various stages of clinical testing; results indicate some curative potential (http://clinicaltrials.gov/ct2/results?cond=%22Macular+Degeneration%22).

control research
Research whose major aim is to control symptoms, not cure the disease or condition. Pain medications control the symptoms of arthritis; they do not cure the underlying disease.

A second type of research is **control research**, designed to reduce the symptoms or severity of the disease. Chemotherapy, heart medications, and thyroid hormone are three examples of controlling diseases. Chemotherapy combined with other treatments may reduce or eliminate the cancer from a body, but often control of the disease process is the major goal. Heart medications control the rate and strength of the heartbeat to improve the person's quality of life, but they do not cure heart disease. Thyroid hormone is given to replace the body's own when the thyroid ceases to function effectively. Although it mimics the original glandular function, it does not cure the processes that destroyed the thyroid or cause it to regenerate. These three treatments are results of research where the goal was to control a process, not cure it. The goal of stem cell and human genome research is to be able to regenerate tissue and make unnecessary the use of thyroid, insulin, antidepressives, and other medications that only control diseases. The ambition is to cure the condition with genetic manipulation.

prevention research
Research whose major aim is to find ways to prevent a disease or condition. For example, preventive research found that diet, exercise, and certain drugs like aspirin may prevent a second heart attack.

The third type of research is **prevention research**, which looks for the causes of a condition or disease and then tries to determine how to keep it from happening. Prevention research can focus on any of four phases. In the first phase, it must be determined what diseases and conditions affect the population. Epidemiologists identify and track diseases. This is the primary responsibility of the CDC. In the second phase, the **vector**, or causative agent, for the diseases is identified. Once what causes the disease is known, the vector can be eliminated or controlled. For example, mosquitoes are the vector for malaria, West Nile disease, and many others. If mosquitoes are eradicated, there is no more malaria. The third phase is to find the predisposing factors that put a person at risk for a disease. These include genetic predispositions (inherited diseases), environmental factors (contaminated water, soil, air), and personal behaviors (e.g., unprotected sex, skydiving, or smoking). The fourth phase is the identification of agents, actions, and behaviors that will most likely prevent the condition. The other three phases have determined that the nicotine and tar in cigarettes cause certain types of lung cancer and predispose the individual to atherosclerosis. The pressing question is how to get people either never to smoke or to stop smoking. After 25 years of research on this subject, the rate of smoking in the late teens and early 20s has dropped by only a few percentage points. Getting large numbers of people to adopt healthy lifestyles is a major area of preventive research.

> **vector** An organism that transmits disease-causing microbes from infected individuals to other persons or from infected animals to human beings. Fleas were the vectors from rats to people in the great plagues.

Funding and the Grant Process

In the United States, the federal government's expenditures for health care research are about $30 billion a year (http://www.nih.gov/about/budget.htm). This does not include the amount spent by state governments in matching grants or state research priorities. Pharmaceutical companies spend approximately the same amount of money in research to generate new drugs each year as the total U.S. government research budget for all types of health care research.

Much more money is spent on the cure and control of disease than on the prevention of disease in the first place. With the ever-increasing cost of health care, this needs to change. Healthy lifestyle behaviors could save billions of dollars each year. It costs much less to give all pregnant women prenatal care than it does to care for one baby with multiple-system problems because the mother did not get prenatal folic acid or had undiagnosed gestational diabetes or toxemia.

Through the Department of Health and Human Services (DHHS), the U.S. government is the largest health research organization in the world. The DHHS oversees 12 different agencies, each of which does some aspect of health care research (see Table 12.2).

When scientists have an idea they wish to investigate, the first step is to apply for a research grant to the appropriate agency. Identifying the appropriate agency is not as easy as it seems. For instance, the NIH alone has 25 different centers. Each center does both primary research on the area of interest and all the types of prevention and health outcomes research (see Table 12.3).

Located in Bethesda, Maryland, the NIH has about 75 buildings on more than 300 acres. These include a clinical research hospital and research center where patients undergoing clinical trials are cared for by NIH staff nurses, physicians, and other health care providers.

Table 12.2	*Departments of Health and Human Services*

Office of the Secretary
Administration for Children and Families
Administration on Aging
Agency for Healthcare Research and Quality
Agency for Toxic Substances and Disease Registry
Centers for Disease Control and Prevention
Centers for Medicare & Medicaid Services
Food and Drug Administration
Health Resources and Services Administration
Indian Health Service
National Institutes of Health
Program Support Center
Substance Abuse and Mental Health Services Administration

Source: http://www.hhs.gov/.

Table 12.3	*National Institutes of Health*

National Cancer Institute (NCI) — Est. 1937
NCI leads a national effort to eliminate the suffering and death due to cancer. Through basic and clinical biomedical research and training, NCI conducts and supports research that will lead to a future in which we can prevent cancer before it starts, identify cancers that do develop at the earliest stage, eliminate cancers through innovative treatment interventions, and biologically control those cancers that we cannot eliminate so they become manageable, chronic diseases.

National Eye Institute (NEI) — Est. 1968
The National Eye Institute's mission is to conduct and support research, training, health information dissemination, and other programs with respect to blinding eye diseases, visual disorders, mechanisms of visual function, preservation of sight, and the special health problems and requirements of the blind.

National Heart, Lung, and Blood Institute (NHLBI) — Est. 1948
The National Heart, Lung, and Blood Institute (NHLBI) provides global leadership for a research, training, and education program to promote the prevention and treatment of heart, lung, and blood diseases and enhance the health of all individuals so that they can live longer and more fulfilling lives. The NHLBI stimulates basic discoveries about the causes of disease, enables the translation of basic discoveries into clinical practice, fosters training and mentoring of emerging scientists and physicians, and communicates research advances to the public.

National Human Genome Research Institute (NHGRI) — Est. 1989
NHGRI is devoted to advancing health through genome research. The Institute led NIH's contribution to the Human Genome Project, which was successfully completed in 2003 ahead of schedule and under budget. Building on the foundation laid by the sequencing of the human genome, NHGRI's work now encompasses a broad range of research aimed at expanding understanding of human biology and improving human health. In addition, a critical part of NHGRI's mission continues to be the study of the ethical, legal, and social implications of genome research.

Table 12.3   *(continued)*

National Institute on Aging (NIA) — Est. 1974
NIA leads a national program of research on the biomedical, social, and behavioral aspects of the aging process; the prevention of age-related diseases and disabilities; and the promotion of a better quality of life for all older Americans.

National Institute on Alcohol Abuse and Alcoholism (NIAAA) — Est. 1970
NIAAA conducts research focused on improving the treatment and prevention of alcoholism and alcohol-related problems to reduce the enormous health, social, and economic consequences of this disease.

National Institute of Allergy and Infectious Diseases (NIAID) — Est. 1948
NIAID research strives to understand, treat, and ultimately prevent the myriad infectious, immunologic, and allergic diseases that threaten millions of human lives.

National Institute of Arthritis and Musculoskeletal and Skin Diseases (NIAMS) — Est. 1986
NIAMS supports research into the causes, treatment, and prevention of arthritis and musculoskeletal and skin diseases, the training of basic and clinical scientists to carry out this research, and the dissemination of information on research progress in these diseases.

National Institute of Biomedical Imaging and Bioengineering (NIBIB) — Est. 2000
The mission of the National Institute of Biomedical Imaging and Bioengineering (NIBIB) is to improve health by leading the development and accelerating the application of biomedical technologies. The Institute is committed to integrating the physical and engineering sciences with the life sciences to advance basic research and medical care.

Eunice Kennedy Shriver National Institute of Child Health and Human Development (NICHD) — Est. 1962
NICHD research on fertility, pregnancy, growth, development, and medical rehabilitation strives to ensure that every child is born healthy and wanted and grows up free from disease and disability.

National Institute on Deafness and Other Communication Disorders (NIDCD) — Est. 1988
NIDCD conducts and supports biomedical research and research training on normal mechanisms as well as diseases and disorders of hearing, balance, smell, taste, voice, speech, and language that affect 46 million Americans.

National Institute of Dental and Craniofacial Research (NIDCR) — Est. 1948
NIDCR provides leadership for a national research program designed to understand, treat, and ultimately prevent the infectious and inherited craniofacial–oral–dental diseases and disorders that compromise millions of human lives.

National Institute of Diabetes and Digestive and Kidney Diseases (NIDDK) — Est. 1950
The mission of the National Institute of Diabetes and Digestive and Kidney Diseases (NIDDK) is to conduct and support medical research and research training and to disseminate science-based information on diabetes and other

(continued)

Table 12.3	*National Institutes of Health (continued)*

endocrine and metabolic diseases; digestive diseases, nutritional disorders, and obesity; and kidney, urologic, and hematologic diseases, to improve people's health and quality of life.

National Institute on Drug Abuse (NIDA) — Est. 1974
NIDA leads the nation in bringing the power of science to bear on drug abuse and addiction through strategic support and conduct of research across a broad range of disciplines and rapid and effective dissemination and use of the results of that research to significantly improve prevention and treatment and to inform policy as it relates to drug abuse and addiction.

National Institute of Environmental Health Sciences (NIEHS) — Est. 1969
The mission of the National Institute of Environmental Health Sciences is to discover how the environment affects people in order to promote healthier lives.

National Institute of General Medical Sciences (NIGMS) — Est. 1962
The National Institute of General Medical Sciences (NIGMS) supports basic research that increases understanding of biological processes and lays the foundation for advances in disease diagnosis, treatment, and prevention. NIGMS-funded scientists investigate how living systems work at a range of levels, from molecules and cells to tissues, whole organisms, and populations. The Institute also supports research in certain clinical areas, primarily those that affect multiple organ systems. To ensure the vitality and continued productivity of the research enterprise, NIGMS provides leadership in training the next generation of scientists, in enhancing the diversity of the scientific workforce, and in developing research capacities throughout the country.

National Institute of Mental Health (NIMH) — Est. 1949
NIMH provides national leadership dedicated to understanding, treating, and preventing mental illnesses through basic research on the brain and behavior, and through clinical, epidemiological, and services research.

National Institute on Minority Health and Health Disparities (NIMHD) — Est. 1993
The mission of NIMHD is to lead scientific research to improve minority health and eliminate health disparities. To accomplish its mission, NIMHD plans, reviews, coordinates, and evaluates all minority health and health disparities research and activities of the National Institutes of Health; conducts and supports research in minority health and health disparities; promotes and supports the training of a diverse research workforce; translates and disseminates research information; and fosters innovative collaborations and partnerships.

National Institute of Neurological Disorders and Stroke (NINDS) — Est. 1950
The mission of NINDS is to seek fundamental knowledge about the brain and nervous system and to use that knowledge to reduce the burden of neurological disease. To accomplish this goal the NINDS supports and conducts basic, translational, and clinical research on the normal and diseased nervous system. The Institute also fosters the training of investigators in the basic and clinical neurosciences and seeks better understanding, diagnosis, treatment, and prevention of neurological disorders.

National Institute of Nursing Research (NINR) — Est. 1986
The mission of the National Institute of Nursing Research (NINR) is to promote and improve the health of individuals, families, communities, and populations.

Table 12.3	*(continued)*

NINR supports and conducts clinical and basic research and research training on health and illness across the life span to build the scientific foundation for clinical practice, prevent disease and disability, manage and eliminate symptoms caused by illness, and improve palliative and end-of-life care.

National Library of Medicine (NLM) — Est. 1956
NLM collects, organizes, and makes available biomedical science information to scientists, health professionals, and the public. The Library's Web-based databases, including PubMed/Medline and MedlinePlus, are used extensively around the world. NLM conducts and supports research in biomedical communications; creates information resources for molecular biology, biotechnology, toxicology, and environmental health; and provides grant and contract support for training, medical library resources, and biomedical informatics and communications research.

A research scientist or team of researchers decides which of the NIH centers is responsible for the research they are interested in and then applies to that institute. Four times a year, the NIH grant screeners receive 10,000 grant applications to review. The research grants may be as small as $50,000 or as large as many millions, depending on what is being researched, how many researchers are involved, and for how long. The standard research grant is for 5 years and can be extended if necessary. Research ideas are funded using a priority system based on the research that identifies the major areas of health care concern in the United States.

For example, a nurse scientist who is interested in the benefits of patient teaching for first-time mothers would apply to the National Institute of Nursing Research (a center of the NIH) for funding for the project. Because there are many requests for grants and few granted, the first step may be to take the NINR research training course. This course takes the new researcher through the steps necessary to write a successful grant. It may take a year to write the grant, then another year to actually get the grant. Then the researcher must report to the NINR each quarter and submit a budget each year. This elaborate process allows the NIH to have a very competitive process for researchers and enough oversight to ensure high-quality research that does not endanger patients or their rights.

An Ounce of Prevention

It has been said that "an apple a day keeps the doctor away." Whether that particular statement is true or not, the focus of prevention is to reduce the amount of health care individuals need.

Prevention research and health goals in the United States are a major focus of both individuals and government agencies. The CDC is the agency charged with tracking health behavior of Americans. But many other agencies and organizations engage in prevention research, tracking, and public service campaigns. The NIH, the Robert Wood Johnson Foundation for health care research, the

Susan B. Komen Foundation for breast cancer, and the American Lung and American Cancer Associations are a few of the leading groups interested in disease prevention and research in the United States.

The leading causes of death are tracked, and programs are instituted to help lessen the impact of these diseases. Table 12.4 lists the major causes of death. When age and gender are taken into account, the leading causes of death in subgroups can vary considerably from this list.

risk factors Anything that contributes to a person getting ill. A feature of someone's habits, genetic history, or personal history that increases the probability he or she will get a particular disease or injury. Smoking is a risk factor for lung cancer.

Many of these causes of death are linked to certain **risk factors** and thus can be changed by changes in behavior. Risk factors such as smoking, high-fat diet, sedentary lifestyle, high blood pressure, elevated cholesterol, obesity, diabetes, and alcohol abuse are linked to the increased incidence of heart disease, cancer, and stroke. The text box provides additional information about the health risks of tobacco use.

Healthy People 2020

health-related quality-of-life (HRQOL) The physical and mental well-being of an individual that looks at the quality and quantity of a healthy life in terms of years.

As you learned at the beginning of this text, according to the CDC's *2014 National Health Survey*, America's health is good overall (61 percent report excellent or very good health), but certain areas need improvement. Based on these survey findings, the DHHS released a document called *Healthy People 2020*, which contains two broad health goals. The first goal is to increase the quality and years of healthy life, and the second is to eliminate health disparities. **Health-related quality of life (HRQOL)** integrates both physical and mental health dimensions so that health is no longer the opposite of disease and death but a concept that stands for well-being (DHHS 2020). *Healthy People 2020* includes 38 areas of focus.

Table 12.4	*Leading Causes of Death in the United States, 2013*

Deaths and Mortality
- Number of deaths: 2,596,993
- Death rate: 821.5 deaths per 100,000 population
- Life expectancy: 78.8 years
- Infant mortality rate: 5.96 deaths per 1,000 live births

Number of deaths for leading causes of death:
- Heart disease: 611,105
- Cancer: 584,881
- Chronic lower respiratory diseases: 149,205
- Accidents (unintentional injuries): 130,557
- Stroke (cerebrovascular diseases): 128,978
- Alzheimer's disease: 84,767
- Diabetes: 75,578
- Influenza and pneumonia: 56,979
- Nephritis, nephrotic syndrome, and nephrosis: 47,112
- Intentional self-harm (suicide): 41,149

Source: http://www.cdc.gov/nchs/fastats/deaths.htm.

Health Risks of Tobacco Use

Tobacco and Disease

- Tobacco use causes—

  Cancer

  Heart disease

  Lung diseases (including emphysema, bronchitis, and chronic airway obstruction)

- Cigarette smoking increases the length of time that people live with a disability by about 2 years.
- For every person who dies from a smoking-related disease, 30 more people suffer with at least one serious illness from smoking.

Tobacco and Death

Worldwide

Tobacco use causes more than 6 million deaths per year.

Current trends show that tobacco use will cause more than 8 million deaths annually by 2030.

On average, smokers die 10 years earlier than nonsmokers.

In the United States

Cigarette smoking is the leading preventable cause of death; more than 16 million Americans have a disease caused by smoking

Cigarette smoking is responsible for about 1 in 5 deaths annually, or about 480,000 deaths per year.

An estimated 41,000 of tobacco-related deaths are the result of secondhand smoke exposure.

Smokers, on average, die 10 years earlier than nonsmokers.

Costs of Smoking

- Annually, in the United States, **cigarette smoking** costs more than $300 billion

in health care expenditures and lost productivity.

- Annually, in the United States, **secondhand smoke** costs more than $10 billion in health care expenditures.

Tobacco Use in the United States

- 42 million people in the United States smoke cigarettes.
- Each day over 5,000 people under the age of 18 either take their first smoke or go from occasional smoker to a daily smoker.
- Each day, approximately 1,800 adults 18 years of age and older become daily smokers (i.e., begin smoking on a daily basis).

Quitting

Many adult smokers want or try to quit smoking:

- Approximately 70 percent of smokers want to quit completely.
- Approximately 42 percent of smokers try to quit each year.

Cessation treatments found to be effective include the following:

- Brief clinical interventions
- Counseling
- Over-the-counter and prescription nicotine replacement products (e.g., nicotine gum, inhaler, nasal spray, lozenge, or patch)
- Prescription nonnicotine medications, such as bupropion SR (Zyban®) and varenicline tartrate (Chantix®)

Source: http://www.cdc.gov/tobacco/data_statistics/fact_sheets/fast_facts/index.htm.

The subjects for prevention campaigns and budget come from these focus areas. Progress has been generally positive toward achieving these targets from 2010 to 2014. Fourteen of the 26 indicators (53.9%) have either met their target or shown improvement. The focus areas are presented in Table 12.5.

Table 12.5	*Healthy People 2020*

Access to Health Services
Adolescent Health
Arthritis, Osteoporosis, and Chronic Back Conditions
Blood Disorders and Blood Safety
Cancer
Chronic Kidney Diseases
Diabetes
Disability and Secondary Conditions
Early and Middle Childhood
Educational and Community-Based Programs
Environmental Health
Family Planning
Food Safety
Genomics
Global Health
Health Communication and Health IT
Healthcare-Associated Infections
Hearing and Other Sensory or Communication Disorders
(Ear, Nose, Throat—Voice, Speech, and Language)
Heart Disease and Stroke
HIV
Immunization and Infectious Diseases
Injury and Violence Prevention
Maternal, Infant, and Child Health
Medical Product Safety
Mental Health and Mental Disorders
Nutrition and Weight Status
Occupational Safety and Health
Older Adults
Oral Health
Physical Activity and Fitness
Public Health Infrastructure
Quality of Life and Well-Being
Respiratory Diseases
Sexually Transmitted Diseases
Social Determinants of Health
Substance Abuse
Tobacco Use
Vision

Source: http://www.healthypeople.gov/2020/leading-health-indicators/Healthy-People-2020-Leading-Health-Indicators%3A-Progress-Update.

The progress made toward these goals was discussed in Chapter 1. Many of the focus areas are influenced by personal behavior patterns. As health care professionals design strategies to improve health, models of behavior such as the Health Promotion Model used in nursing can be helpful. The model has three components: individual characteristics, behavior-specific cognitions and affect, and behavioral outcomes (Pender, Murdaugh, and Parsons 2013). Without understanding the influence of the first two components, the final step of health-promoting behavior is unlikely to occur.

The NIH has affirmed that different strategies are needed at different ages and genders. For children, health promotion should include routine infant screenings, immunizations, instruction to caregivers on accident prevention and proper diet and exercise, and dental care. Adolescents as a group are very healthy, but many unhealthy practices, such as smoking, substance abuse, and unprotected sex, begin at this time. Promotion activities should focus on education.

Health promotion for adult men and women is quite different, primarily because of reproductive health issues. The strategies for an aging population differ significantly from those of middle-age adults. For women, family planning and prenatal care are essential, as are detection and prevention of unique cancers such as breast cancer and osteoporosis. Although men are at risk for all the causes of death listed in Table 12.4, prostate cancer applies only to men. Men are also at much higher risk for violence.

The health of older adults is an increasing concern given the overall aging of the population and increased longevity. Poor nutrition and vision and hearing problems are particularly acute in this population. Accident prevention is essential because falls can contribute to a host of other, more severe health problems.

Women's Health

Women's health is one of the areas in which the least progress has been made toward the *Healthy People 2020 goals*, according to the CDC:

- 85% of women under 65 have some sort of health insurance, a major increase since the Affordable Care Act implementation.
- 14% of women over the age of 18 rate their health as poor or fair.
- 16% of adult women smoke.
- 36% of women are obese.
- 33% of women over 20 have clinical hypertension and are taking medication.
- 69% of women over 18 have a Pap smear every 3 years.
- 67% of women over 40 have a mammogram every 2 years.
- Leading causes of death among women—all are related to smoking, obesity and lack of exercise, and hypertension:
  - Heart disease
  - Cancer
  - Chronic respiratory disease
- Only 17 states provide women with safe abortion procedures.

Because many women and at least one in every four children in the United States live in poverty, access to care will remain a social, political, and health problem for years to come.

We know how to prevent or mitigate many diseases, but we do not know how to ensure that women and men who need basic health care get it. If we cannot meet the first focus on healthy people, it is unlikely that significant gains will be made on the other goals, which all require access to health care to implement.

The current debate on health care offers a unique opportunity to focus on reproductive health. The average woman spends 5 of the 35 years of fertility having children and 30 years trying not to get pregnant. It takes a healthy woman to have a healthy baby. The need for increased access to reproductive health care is demonstrated by the high rate of unintended pregnancies, low birth weight and neurologically impaired babies, increased maternal diabetes and hypertension, increased sexually transmitted diseases (STDs) in all age groups, and inadequate access to breast care and uterine/cervical cancer screening. The United States does not have a seamless continuum of care that addresses preconception, pregnancy planning, birth spacing, emergency contraception, post-natal care, and general reproductive health. We also lack a health care delivery system that integrates reproductive health into primary care delivery for either women or men. For many women, primary care in the reproductive years may be delivered by a variety of health care providers—physicians (MDs and ODs), nurse practitioners, complementary medicine providers, and both certified and lay midwives, which increases the fragmentation of care for women.

The Business Response for Prevention

Corporations and insurance companies are as concerned about improving health as the federal government is. Data consistently indicate that prevention lowers health care costs and increases productivity (Surgeon General 2011). Increasing insurance costs, government mandates, and lost productivity affect businesses directly, leading them to take a proactive role in health education and promotion.

According to the CDC, between 75 and 85 percent of health care spending in the United States was for people with one or more chronic conditions, such as heart disease, stroke, cancer, diabetes, and obesity. One estimate is that obesity and related chronic diseases cost employers about $93 billion in health insurance claims (www.cdc.gov/features/workingwellness/). In addition to direct costs, the indirect costs of poor health such as absenteeism and reduced work output may be several times higher than the direct cost of insurance payments. Sometimes, the absenteeism is related to an employee who provides caregiving to the person with a chronic illness.

In addition to reducing these direct and indirect costs, employers can utilize workplace programs as a recruiting and retention tool. Companies like Google,

Safeway, and PepsiCo improve their reputations as good places to work because of the programs they offer.

A workplace health program is an activity or policy designed to support healthy behaviors and improve health outcomes while at work. This can include health education and coaching, weight management programs, medical screenings, and on-site fitness facilities. Employers can design policies to change the work environment to encourage health, including allowing time for exercise during work hours, providing on-site kitchens and eating areas, and providing healthy options in vending machines. Some companies have even moved to "walk and talk" meetings. In order to encourage participation, employers offer financial and other incentives (www.cdc.gov/workplacehealthpromotion). The Affordable Care Act allows employers to offer 30 to 50 percent reductions in health coverage costs as an incentive. Thus far, large companies have been more likely to implement programs than small companies or public-sector employers.

Clearly businesses and their insurance companies have a huge financial incentive to help employees improve their health. The question that isn't clear is which programs return the most benefit for the least cost. Organizations such as the Wellness Council of America (www.welcoa.org) have studied workplace programs for more than 20 years; WELCOA estimates that for every $1 spent on wellness programs, the employer saves $3 in health insurance costs. The CDC recommends that employers study their health care data, and survey employees to decide which programs would be most valuable. Employers can reach out to a number of organizations and to state health organizations to obtain assistance in creating programs (www.cdc.gov/workplacehealthpromotion/organizations/index.htm). The CDC warns that as employees become more educated about the benefits of preventive health care tools such as screenings, a company might see an initial spike in its health care costs. However, this should pay off in the longer term, both in a healthier workforce and in terms of employee satisfaction.

The Individual's Response for Prevention

Americans have more access to health information than ever before. Table 12.6 lists just a few of the many sources of health information; a simple Google search will find many more. The increasing number of smartphone apps for health and wellness allow individuals to track their calorie intake, the number of steps they've taken, and the nutritional content of the foods they purchase. Legislative mandates such as those in the Affordable Care Act require that vending machines and chain restaurants post nutritional information about the food they sell. Despite the increased amount of information available, one concern is that those people who need information the most—the poor or uninsured—are also the groups least likely to use the Internet as a health resource.

Data indicate that physical activity can improve many of the health conditions listed in Table 12.4. According to the 2013 National Health Survey, only

Table 12.6	*Sources of Health Information*
General health information	
National Institutes of Health	http://www.nih.gov/
MedlinePlus	medlineplus.gov
Selected topics	
Alzheimer's disease	http://www.nia.nih.gov/alzheimers
American Council on Exercise	www.acefitness.org/default.aspx
Cancer	http://www.cancer.gov/ and www.cancer.net
Children's health	www.kidshealth.org
Family health	www.familydoctor.org
Food and nutrition	www.choosemyplate.gov/
Mayo Clinic	www.mayoclinic.com
Risk assessment	www.YourDiseaseRisk.wustl.edu
Women's health	www.womenshealth.gov; www.hrsa.gov/womenshealth; orwh.od.nih.gov

21 percent of adults regularly engage in physical activity, although this rate varies by age. However, an increased emphasis on fitness has created an entire industry in the last several decades. Fitness industry revenues total almost $24.1 billion, with a total payroll of $7.8 billion. More than 605,000 people are employed by the industry, at 29,682 businesses (U.S. Census Bureau 2012). Fitness centers are available at work; in hospitals; in hotel/motels; on military bases; at schools, colleges, and universities; and at apartment complexes, in addition to commercial health clubs. Both the number of clubs and members have increased; the more than 34,000 health clubs in the United States have more than 54.1 million members (http://clubindustry.com/studies).

Without exercise, prevention of obesity is very difficult in a fast-food culture. Many fast-food choices contain excessive amounts of fat, sodium, and calories. Nutritional information is available from all fast-food companies, making it is possible to eat selections with a better nutritional profile. Many companies are responding to consumer interest in more healthful eating by reducing the amount of fat and sodium (Boston Market, General Mills), removing artificial additives and colors (General Foods, Nestle, Taco Bell, Pizza Hut, Panera Bread), and restricting antibiotics in meat (Chick-fil-A, McDonald's). However, the data are mixed on whether consumers will purchase these healthier options in sufficient numbers to improve their health and improve the companies' profitability.

Prevention alone cannot eradicate disease, but it can reduce the impact of most diseases and make functional, if not clinical, cure a possibility. In conclusion, an apple a day may keep the doctor away, but a good education and income will keep disease at bay.

Career Profile: Health Education Specialists

Helping people learn to be healthier is a growing field of employment. To achieve the *Healthy People 2020* goals, federal, state, and community health organizations have invested heavily in health promotion and prevention activities. These range from boot camp for expectant fathers to antismoking campaigns subsidized by the states' tobacco tax. Major program areas include smoking and health, breast and cervical cancer prevention, diabetes disability prevention, HIV/AIDS prevention, and school health education. Whatever the activity, it is planned and implemented by a health education specialist.

Health education specialists consult with state and local health officials on chronic disease prevention and health promotion. They are involved in strategic planning, program implementation, monitoring, and evaluation of programs. They work with ethnically and racially diverse groups, which requires an understanding of and ability to communicate effectively with these groups. Health education specialists can be found working in a wide variety of organizations including the CDC, the military, hospitals, public health, community health, city and state agencies, and fitness centers.

The basic requirement is a 4-year degree in health education, education, or related field from an accredited college. Your education should include at least 24 credit hours in health education or education and appropriate course work in health. Most positions then require at least 1 year of work experience as a paid intern or volunteer externship in a health education setting. The salaries range from $33,000 to $50,000 for those with a bachelor's degree. Those with a doctorate and director-level responsibilities could earn as much as $150,000. This means there is a solid career ladder with opportunity for upward growth.

Summary

Health care research and prevention are two ways to minimize the impact of disease on the population. Research can focus on three goals: cure, control, or prevention. Research scientists work in many settings: universities, companies, not-for-profits, and the government. The federal government is the largest sponsor of health care research. The CDC tracks disease and death rates to help formulate and implement programs to prevent or lessen the impact of disease. Personal behavior patterns, such as nutrition, smoking, exercise, weight control, and regular screening, promote healthy outcomes. Access to care is a major determinant of health; income and education are major predictors of access to health care. Women have less access to health care than men and as a result have lower health status.

Questions for Review

1. Give examples of the three major types of research.
2. Describe the function and scope of the Department of Health and Human Services.
3. What is the NIH, and what does it do?

4. Describe the process of obtaining a research grant from the NIH.
5. How does the government decide which research projects to fund?
6. How is the flu vaccine determined each year?
7. What is the status of women's and workplace health goals for *Healthy People 2020*?
8. What incentives can businesses offer to impact wellness?

Questions for Discussion

1. What is your experience with the flu vaccine?
   a. Do you get a yearly flu shot? Why? Why not?
   b. Have you had the flu in the last 5 years?
   c. Survey the class: How many have had the flu? The flu shots? How does that compare to the national average?
2. Using a government website, describe the research being done on one of the top 10 causes of death.
3. In your opinion, what method should be used to determine the subjects of health care research? Using your method you've chosen, what types of research would be supported?
4. Describe the steps being taken to reach the goal of one of the objectives of *Healthy People 2020*.
5. At your school or place of work, what tools are available to help you take care of yourself?
6. Go to the websites of several fast-food companies to access nutritional information. How do your favorites compare?
7. How does your state rank in meeting the *Healthy People 2020* goals?
8. How would you determine your own health status using assessment tools on the Web?

Chapter References

https://www.aids.gov/hiv-aids-basics/hiv-aids-101/global-statistics/
http://www.aphis.usda.gov/wps/portal/aphis/ourfocus/animalhealth/sa_animal_disease_information/sa_avian_health/ct_avian_influenza_disease
http://www.cdc.gov/flu/about/season/flu-season-2015-2016.htm
http://www.cdc.gov/flu/about/season/index.htm
http://www.cdc.gov/nchs/data/series/sr_10/sr10_260.pdf
http://www.cdc.gov/nchs/fastats/womens-health.htm
http://www.cdc.gov/nchs/data/hus/hus14.pdf#001
http://www.cdc.gov/nchs/data/nhis/earlyrelease/earlyrelease201406.pdf
http://www.cdc.gov/nchs/data/hus/hus14.pdf#054
http://www.cdc.gov/nchs/data/hus/hus14.pdf#064
http://www.cdc.gov/nchs/data/hus/hus14.pdf#060
http://www.cdc.gov/nchs/data/hus/hus14.pdf#076
http://www.cdc.gov/employment/menu_topjobs.html#HealthEdSpcs

http://www.cdc.gov/nchs/data/nvsr/nvsr64/nvsr64_02.pdf

Clinical Trials: http://clinicaltrials.gov/ct2/results?cond=%22Macular+
Degeneration%22

Flu.Gov (www.flu.gov).

http://www.hhs.gov/

National Center for Health Statistics. 2015. *Health, United States, 2014: With special feature
on adults aged 55–64.* Hyattsville, MD: Author.

National Institute of Allergy and Infectious Disease (http://www.niaid.nih.gov/
factsheets/flu.htm).

http://www.opm.gov/policy-data-oversight/pay-leave/salaries-wages/salary-tables/
pdf/2014/POR.pdf

Pender, N., C. Murdaugh, and M. Parsons. 2013. *Health promotion in nursing.* 6th ed.
Upper Saddle River, NJ: Prentice Hall.

Surgeon General. 2011. National Prevention Strategy, Appendix 1. http://www.
surgeongeneral.gov/priorities/prevention/strategy/report.pdf

U.S. Census Bureau. 2012. *2012 Economic Census, Industry series reports. NAICS 713940.*

For Additional Information

Genetics Home Reference (http://ghr.nlm.nih.gov/).

See any of the websites listed in Table 12.6.

13

Cultural Competency, Health Literacy, and Health Care Ethics

Learning Objectives

After reading this chapter, you should be able to:

1. Define cultural competency.
2. Describe REALM.
3. Explain the ideal of health literacy.
4. Identify the benefits of health and cultural literacy to the country.
5. Assess your own and your family's health literacy.
6. Discuss and give examples of four health literacy strategies.
7. Discuss ethical issues in cultural competency theories.
8. Identify and describe three major ethical theories.
9. Identify four major ethical principles in health care.
10. Discuss the ethical rationale for health care reform.

Pima Indians and Diabetes

Sadie is a member of the Pima Indian tribe of the Gila River Indian Community. Her ancestors were among the first people to set foot in the Americas 30,000 years ago. They have lived in the Sonoran Desert near the Gila River in what is now southern Arizona for at least 2,000 years.

What makes the Pima Indian tribe very special in modern medical history is that they have participated in one of the longest-running research projects of the Indian Health Service. For the last 30 years, members of this tribe have been studied, have taken surveys, and have had every aspect of their lives described by researchers. The reason for the interest? Over 50 percent of all adult Pima tribe members have Type II—adult diabetes and at a very young age, usually by 36. In comparison, about 8 percent of the general population in the 20 to 60 age group has Type II diabetes, rising to about 23 percent by age 60. In addition, the tribe's diabetics have a much greater risk of having Kidney Disease of Diabetes Mellitus (KDDM) and kidney failure. The community is the smallest town (population 1,100) in the United States with its own kidney dialysis center. In contrast, the national rate was 9 percent with Native Americans at 15.9 percent in 2012. The Pima tribe had an epidemic of diabetes.

The sand-colored stucco home where Sadie lives with her husband and three daughters in Gila is neat as a pin. Her household chores are good exercise, she says, to help control her own diabetes. Sadie's mother, who developed diabetes shortly after her daughter was born, died from kidney disease that developed from her long-term diabetes. Her father, a retired heavy equipment operator who had been very active in reservation life, suffered an amputation—a complication of his diabetes—a year ago, after being hospitalized for several long months. "He got a sore on his foot and never got it treated," she explains. Four of her 10 brothers and sisters also have the disease, which runs in families. Although she has seen the worst diabetes can do, Sadie is not giving up. What her father and other family members have gone through makes her want to take care of herself: "I could be in that same situation."

She is also motivated by wanting to see her three daughters, aged 12, 7, and 3, keep their health. All were big babies, and they have remained heavy for their ages. "All of my kids are chubby," she adds. That's common for babies born to mothers who have or are prone to develop diabetes, according to NIH researchers who are studying the disease in the Pima Indians. This mother is trying to teach her daughters to watch what they eat because being overweight increases dramatically the risk of diabetes.

Introduction

The study of ethics and cultural competency in the health care arena originates from the idea that there should be fairness and equality in the delivery of health care benefits. This chapter deals with the institutional issues in health care ethics, rather than the individual case. The same holds true for our discussion of cultural competency: it is not so much being able to talk to a single individual; but to achieve fairness and equality, it is critical to have organizational and institutional tools in place that allow the providers to talk to people at all levels of health literacy.

Her third grader, a pretty child with glossy black hair who likes to read when she isn't playing with her cat, already has diabetes. Her mother helps her monitor her blood sugar and is teaching her about choosing healthy foods, although she admits it's hard. When sweets are sometimes given out at school, her daughter gets a toy instead. "I tell her the cookies are gone, but you've still got the toy," her mother says.

Researchers do not yet fully understand why American Indians, and especially the Pima Indians, are more likely to develop diabetes, but one thing is clear—those who are overweight are at high risk. Approximately 95 percent of all Pima Indians and 80 percent of all other people with diabetes are overweight (http://diabetes.niddk.nih.gov/dm/pubs/statistics/). Although researchers are still searching for the genes that cause diabetes in many Pima families, they say that cutting fat in the diet and exercising are the best ways yet known to prevent diabetes and modify its long-term effects (http://www.diabetes.niddk.nih.gov/DM/pubs/pima).

"What I really want to do is change the way we eat here," Sadie explains, referring to fried foods and the tacos the family loves. She knows that eating less sugar and fat is important for her family's health. "They say if you bake or broil, it's supposed to be better, and I've been trying to do that lately."

The need to communicate health care information in a culturally effective and caring way to Sadie and the rest of her tribe led to the Indian Health Service health literacy and cultural competency project. This project uses tools designed to improve communication between the health care provider and the tribal member in a respectful and effective way. Because many tribal members are not health literate, have no access to the Internet, and are very wary of abandoning tribal customs and tribal healers, a new approach was needed. The research on cultural competency demonstrated that there were tools that would help Sadie and her family understand and accept the information needed to care for their diabetic family member. REALM (Rapid Estimate of Adult Literacy in Medicine) is one such tool. We will explore others in this chapter.

Sadie's children and grandchildren have a much better chance to live without diabetes through the efforts of the Indian Health Service's Health Literacy and Cultural Competence programs.

Source: Adapted from http://diabetes.niddk.nih.gov/DM/pubs/pima.

Culture and Health Care

Variables such as age, gender, ethnicity, and socioeconomic status are strongly related to the level of actual and perceived health within a given population. Culture and cultural values are also related to beliefs about health and illness.

Although there are different definitions of culture, social scientists agree that **culture** is learned and shared by group members. What you believe, your values, and much of your behavior are culturally determined. Sociologist Robin Williams has identified 12 **core values** of the American culture: individualism,

culture An integrated and shared pattern of human behavior.

core values Values are shared attitudes and beliefs among group members. Core values are the central values of a culture.

freedom, democracy, equality, achievement and success, efficiency and practicality, progress, science and technology, material comfort, activity and work, humanitarianism, and group superiority (Henslin 2014). Definitions are presented in Table 13.1. However, these values are constantly being changed and challenged as the ethnic landscape and generational adoption of social media and communication evolve.

Table 13.1	*Cultural Values in America*
Individualism	Americans believe that individual effort and initiative lead to success. If a person doesn't get ahead, it's his fault.
Freedom	Americans resent any limitation on their personal freedom. Even though Americans are widely aware of the dangers of unhealthy choices such as drinking, smoking, and overeating, they resist any attempt to regulate those behaviors, believing even bad choices to be an individual's right.
Democracy	Americans believe that everyone has the right to express an opinion and that the majority rules.
Equality	Equal opportunity is an ideal of American society.
Achievement and success	Personal achievement is highly valued and is measured by attaining wealth, power, and prestige. For this reason, many people respect physicians.
Efficiency and practicality	Doing things as efficiently as possible and making changes to improve efficiency are considered strengths.
Progress	Americans expect technology to change rapidly.
Science and technology	Americans develop new technology and expect science to control natural forces. If a new disease is identified (e.g., AIDS or SARS), Americans expect scientists to find a cure quickly.
Material comfort	Americans expect to be comfortable. Americans take over-the-counter medications and expect their health care services to be relatively pain free.
Activity and work	Even when not at work, Americans expect people to be "busy." Leisure activities such as sports and exercise are good behaviors.
Humanitarianism	Americans value helpfulness and kindness. They volunteer and contribute to many health-related groups such as the American Cancer Society. In times of mass disasters, they provide aid individually or through the Red Cross and other organizations.
Group superiority	Despite the values of equality and democracy, American have valued some groups more highly than others. In its ugliest form, this value has been expressed as racism.

Source: Henslin 2014.

Often these values come into conflict. For example, Americans value both efficiency and humanitarianism. Therefore, many Americans are dissatisfied with a health care system that treats them efficiently but does not take time to recognize them as individuals. Others view the current system as one that is inherently unjust because the system does not treat people equally. As we will explore, women, people of color, and the poor all have issues with health care in the United States.

Of course, in a country as large as the United States there are also subcultures. **Subcultures** are groups that share many of the elements of mainstream culture, but maintain their own distinctive customs, values, norms, and lifestyles. Subcultures can be based on gender, age, ethnicity, religion, sexual preference, and occupation, to name just a few variables. Occupations such as health care and places of employment such as hospitals can be considered as subcultures because they have their own specialized language, customs, and material culture.

Disease and illness occur within a cultural context, even to the extent of defining what is and is not a disease. Some of the aspects of culture that affect health care are identified in Table 13.2.

The United States has five ethnic minority groups—Native Americans/ Alaskan Native, Hispanics/Latina, Asian, Native Hawaiian, and African American. Data indicate that these cultures have different health outcomes from the dominant white culture. In addition, they have different health practices and access health care differently. A challenge for the health care industry is to ensure that all Americans receive good quality care.

One consequence of culture is that our culture influences the way we see the world. However, as the United States becomes more diverse culturally, it is more common to encounter people of other cultures. As an example of this increasing diversity, in one of my recent classes in Health Care Management, seven different languages were spoken, and the students represented four continents. If a person is **ethnocentric**, he or she will evaluate others' customs according to values of his or her own cultural group. This can lead to misperceptions and conflict. Anne Fadiman's account of an epileptic Hmong child's interaction with the U.S. health care system illustrates how vastly different cultures and their perceptions of illness can come into conflict (Fadiman 1997). The U.S. system viewed epilepsy as a disease that needed treatment, whereas the Hmong parents viewed the seizures as evidence of visits by spirits.

subculture A group within a main culture that accepts the standards of the main culture, but has distinctive customs and values.

ethnocentrism The evaluation of behaviors according to one's own cultural beliefs.

Table 13.2	*Aspects of Culture That Impact Health Care*
Language	Beliefs about health and illness
Time orientation	Beliefs about aging
Family practices	Death practices
Childbirth practices	Pain response
Child-rearing practices	Grief response
Food habits	Touch and privacy
Sexuality	

Ethnocentrism can also affect relations between health care businesses and their employees.

Culture affects how people communicate, understand, and respond to health information. Cultural and linguistic competency of health professionals contributes to health literacy. **Health literacy** is defined as the degree to which individuals have the capacity to obtain, process, and understand basic information and services needed to make appropriate decisions about their health. Culture refers to integrated patterns of human behavior that include the language, thoughts, communications, actions, customs, beliefs, values, and institutions of racial, ethnic, religious, gender, age, or social groups. Competence implies having the capacity to function effectively as an individual and an organization within the context of the cultural beliefs, behaviors, and needs presented by consumers and their communities.

health literacy The degree to which individuals have the capacity to obtain, process, and understand basic information and services needed to make appropriate decisions about their health.

Cultural competence is the ability of health organizations and practitioners to recognize the cultural beliefs, values, attitudes, traditions, language preferences, and health practices of specific cultural groups and to apply that knowledge to produce positive health outcomes. Competency includes communicating in a manner that is linguistically and culturally appropriate. Health care professionals have their own culture and language (http://www11.georgetown.edu/research/gucchd/nccc/foundations/frameworks).

cultural competence The ability of health organizations and practitioners to recognize cultural beliefs, values, attitudes, traditions, language preferences, and health practices of specific cultural groups and to apply that knowledge to produce positive health outcomes.

Many adopt the "culture of medicine" and the language of their specialty as a result of their training and work environment. This can affect how health professionals communicate with the public. If the patient is health literate, he or she will have the ability to understand health care providers' information such as prescription instructions, disease brochures, and health care instructions. Health literacy is not dependent on the ability to read, but rather to understand what is said to patients regardless of their culture, reading ability, or language (http://www.minorityhealth.hhs.gov).

Why Are Cultural Competence and Health Literacy Important?

Cultural competency and health literacy are two of the main ingredients in closing the gap in the disparity of health care services provided to different groups. It's the way patients and health care providers can come together and talk about health concerns so that cultural differences can enhance rather than hinder the conversation. Health care services that are respectful of and responsive to the health beliefs, practices, and cultural and linguistic needs of diverse patients can help bring about positive health outcomes. Research suggests that those who are not health literate experience almost 40 percent more hospitalizations than their health literate counterparts (http://www.ihs.gov/healthcommunications). Culture and language may influence:

- Health, healing, and wellness belief systems
- How illness, disease, and their causes are perceived, by both the patient/consumer and the health care provider

■ The behaviors of patients/consumers who are seeking health care and their attitudes toward health care providers.

The increasing population growth of racial and ethnic communities and linguistic groups, each with its own cultural traits and health profiles, presents a challenge to the health care delivery service in this country. It is estimated that over 90 million people in the United States are not health literate. The provider and the patient each bring their individual learned patterns of language and culture to the health care experience, which must be transcended to achieve equal access and quality health care. All groups who are seen as or perceived to be minorities are affected by cultural competency and health literacy issues. In addition to the five major groups listed, women, children, and elders are also affected (http://bioethics.od.nih.gov/culturalcomp.html):

■ African Americans
■ American Indians/Alaska natives
■ Asian Americans
■ Hispanic/Latinos
■ Native Hawaiians
■ Women
■ Children
■ Elders

We measure the degree to which the group is affected by health literacy and cultural issues by looking at the outcomes of specific diseases and health markers as demonstrated by the profile of the Pima Indians. Some of those markers include the level of access to health care, the level of infant and maternal health, and the status of women's health. Other markers include the status of oral health in the population, the number and type of immunizations, and the level of organ donation. The incidence of certain diseases and health issues, such as asthma, cancer, chronic liver disease, diabetes, hepatitis, HIV/AIDS, obesity, and stroke, are also markers.

How Are Health Care Providers Trained in Cultural Competency and Health Literacy?

Thanks to projects like the Indian Health Service's work with the Pima and other Indian tribes and the Hmong, several tools have been developed to assess and increase cultural competency and health care literacy. One of the most important factors is the ability to use systems already in place in groups to help health providers. In the Pima group, the Healers and Elders were major players in outlining the strategies for intervention in diabetes. Knowing the cultural norms, expectations, fears, and customs of the tribes allowed researchers to develop tools for health care providers.

Health care providers who are working with specific populations need a good orientation to the customs and beliefs of the group, access to language assistance, and a way to rapidly assess health care literacy and appropriate communication tools. To get someone like Sadie to change her family's diet requires culturally appropriate teaching and communication skills as well as the very practical guides to diet and exercise.

Tools Used to Assess and Improve Health Literacy

It is important to clarify a couple of issues about health literacy. First, health literacy is not the same thing as regular literacy. The health care profession has its own language, medical terminology. For those of you who have taken classes in medical terminology, you know that it takes hard study to learn all the concepts of this language and culture. So it is not surprising that people who have not had this training often find what health care providers say hard to understand. Second, many of the groups are not English language proficient—they come from other countries or parts of this country where English is not the first language. They will need to have language appropriate communication, which does not mean just translating medical terminology into another language. A guide to talking with patients provided by the indian Health Service suggests the following:

How to Talk to Patients of Different Cultures and Languages

When talking to patients about their health care issues, remember that patients may be anxious, worried, distressed, and/or confused. Following are a few tips:

- Avoid using technical words or jargon. It may be tough to avoid "physician-speak," but experts say you should assume that all your patients will be confused by most of what you say. If you must use a technical word, define it.

- Avoid unnecessary details. Limit the information you cover in order to reduce confusion or information overload. Use simple vocabulary and short sentences. Make no more than two or three key points for each topic.

- Avoid acronyms. When you must use an acronym, explain the meaning the first time you use it.

- Use the "teach-back" method. Avoid asking patients, "Do you understand?" Most will say they do even when they are confused. Instead say, "I want to make sure I did a good job teaching you. Tell me how you are going to do this when you get home." Research consistently shows that this type of "teach-back" method improves recall and participation in the treatment plan.

- Use pictures. Illustrations often convey instructions better than words.

- Talk to family members. If you think your patient may have low health literacy, enlist the aid of a family member or friend.

Source: http://www.ihs.gov/healthcommunications/index.cfm?module=dsp_hc_toolkit.

The Indian Health Service has developed tools to assist the health care provider to assess health literacy in many different populations. A number of cues may be suggestive of low health literacy status. These cues can include the following:

- Hand brochure to patient upside down and see if he or she correctly aligns the page in order to read it.
- Ask the patient if the print is clear enough to read on the brochure.
- Registration and other forms may be filled out incompletely or incorrectly.
- Patient gives excuses when asked to read something (i.e., forgot reading glasses).
- Patient hands medical brochures/materials to a relative or other person.
- Patient cannot describe how to take medications.

Another tool is the REALM (Rapid Estimate of Adult Literacy in Medicine). This tool asks patients to read and pronounce common medical terms. It has been used to assess health literacy among many different patient populations.

These tools must be used with care and compassion, or they can actually discourage patients from accessing care, much the same way you would be nervous about a quiz (http://www.ihs.gov/healthcommunications).

Ethical Issues in Health Care

The enactment of the Medicare-Medicaid and the End-Stage Renal Disease bills in 1965 fundamentally changed the distribution of health care in the United States from a transaction between the health care provider and the patient to an institutional form of government-mediated health care delivery. This made the federal government the largest broker of health care in the world. The enactment of these two bills entitled large specific segments of the population to the social benefits of health care and thus obligated the federal government to provide those benefits in a fair and just manner. So one could argue that the real beginning of health care ethics as a major area of study and policy was in 1965. Coincidentally, this time period was one of great advances in medical technology and drug therapy. We could now keep people alive through the use of ventilators, pacemakers, and modern surgery. So the question became almost immediately—how does society decide who should get these new benefits and who will be left out? These are the major questions of health care ethics.

Because health care concerns human beings' physical and mental well-being, discussions about health care often contain a lot of "shoulds": "the government should provide basic health care" or "the drug companies should keep drug prices low." In those discussions, a decision about the allocation of scarce resources is based on an ethical viewpoint of how the world should be organized. Health care ethical theories provide a framework to assist patients, health care providers, and policy makers in making these types of decisions.

Ethical issues are those issues in which there are competing values or goods. In an ethical dilemma, there is always more than one answer. This is because both or all the options have some good in them. For example, caring for the elderly is a good. Caring for children is also a good. An ethical dilemma arises when there are insufficient resources to care for both, and choices must be made.

Health care ethics addresses large concepts such as respect for autonomy, nonmaleficence (do no harm), beneficence (do good), justice, veracity (truth telling), privacy, confidentiality, and professional roles. Justice is the major concept used in discussing societal obligations in distributing the health care and will be covered last and in the most detail. The other concepts or principles discussed here are primarily used in the discussion of individual ethical dilemmas and help health care providers and families to talk about ethical decisions they must make on an individual basis.

Autonomy comes from the Greek *auto* (self) and *nomos* (rule)—self-rule. Respect for autonomy requires the health care provider to adhere to the patient's decisions. This concept is the basis for our ideas of informed consent, cultural competence, disclosure of risks, and surrogate decision making. The opposite of autonomy is paternalism—literally the father knows best, or in our context of health care—the health care provider knows what is best for the patient.

Nonmaleficence, a technical philosophical term, requires health care providers not to inflict harm intentionally or simply put—at least do no harm. Many bioethical controversies involve the principle of do no harm. Policy makers in states like Oregon had to balance the patient's right of autonomy against the health care providers' mandate to do no harm in the Death with Dignity legislation. Many court cases have revolved around the giving or withholding life-sustaining treatment, again an ethical dilemma involving patient/family wishes and the health care providers' perspective. These are large questions, which involve the patients and their health care providers, but also the public, policy makers, the courts, and legislators.

Beneficence requires us to contribute positively to the welfare of others—do good, not evil. It continues the idea of do no harm into a demand to provide benefits. This principle is expressed when we talk about the government's role in providing public health or when we talk about the need to balance the cost of a program with the benefits it will give to people. The Good Samaritan Rule is a good example of beneficence: you should stop at a wreck and provide first aid if you are able. You are giving a positive benefit to the injured person. Some states have legislated beneficence so that health care providers with basic first aid are required to either stop and help or report injuries. Further legislation has protected the person acting under the Good Samaritan Rule from lawsuits, an expression that the good it does to have people help those who are injured outweighs some legal rights.

Codes of ethics are based on a combination of the concepts just mentioned and the idea that health care professionals are held to a higher ethical standard than nonprofessionals.

These codes of ethics demand a certain standard of behavior if one is to be in good standing with the health care professions. They are universal principles that are required of health care professionals in every aspect of health care from physicians to the scientist and medical records clerk and everyone in between. The major principles involved in professional behavior are veracity (telling the truth) and confidentiality. Along with the virtues of compassion, integrity, trustworthiness, and wisdom, these principles guide the health care professional in the care of patients.

Justice and the Health Care System

The principle of justice is probably the most often quoted principle when people talk about health care reform or the government's role in public health. The terms *fairness* and *entitlement* are frequently used in those conversations that discuss allocation of resources. We use theories of justice to help decide how to distribute fairly the benefits of society. These theories were devised because simple ideas of justice do not work well on the macro scale of society. We cannot just divide health care equally among all citizens because some need more and some don't need any at all. So the pie is unequal from the beginning.

There are several major ethical theories used to help health policy makers and governments divide the pie. These include **rights theory, utilitarianism,** and **Kantian**, to name a few. Those theories are studied in an ethics, bioethics, or business ethics class in a much greater degree than is possible in this brief overview.

All these theories have been used to examine the issues of health care in the United States. Policy decisions about health care make trade-offs between three competing "shoulds":

1. **Access:** As many people as possible should be able to receive health care services.
2. **Quality:** The health care services should be of the highest possible quality.
3. **Cost:** The health care services should not cost too much.

These three policy drivers or shoulds are presented in Figure 13.1. What policy makers usually discover is that they can achieve one or two of these objectives, but that they cannot simultaneously achieve all three. Ethical theories can provide a rationale and framework for these difficult choices.

In rights theory, health care is viewed as a basic human and citizen right. Rights theory and the principle of justice were the primary rationales for the Patient Protection and Affordable Care Act of 2010. The argument was that health care was a right of all citizens, not the few who could pay or belong to special groups, and therefore the government had an obligation to provide basic health care for all. Prior to the Affordable Care Act, only special groups such as the over-65 age group or veterans had a right to health care. Although the Affordable Care Act did not mandate health care as a right of all citizens, the act considerably expanded access through its regulation of health insurance. All rights under this theory have a companion obligation.

The utilitarian theory revolves around the idea that health care resources should be allocated where they will do the most good. This would suggest some sort of a rationing of health care so that the neediest would always get health care.

rights theory An ethical theory that believes people have certain basic rights as human beings and as citizens.

utilitarianism An ethical theory that believes resources should be distributed to achieve the maximum benefit.

Kantian theory An ethical theory developed by Immanuel Kant (1724–1804) that says a universal moral law obligates one to treat people as an end in itself.

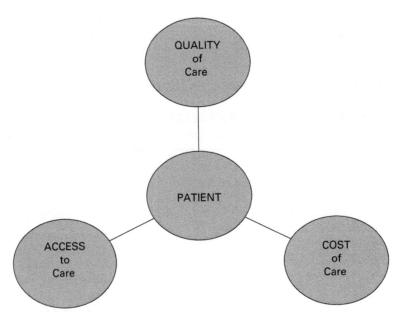

Figure 13.1   Policy Trade-Offs

John Stuart Mill first introduced this theory in the 19th century. He proposed that moral decisions should be made on the basis of the most good for the most people. In terms of social policy, his theory is a long-term project, not just a simple equation. The health care systems of Britain, Scandinavia, and Canada reflect the utilitarian idea that health care is a good, and having the most people have access to the system is a societal good that must be shared according to the individual's, need for it, regardless of the person's ability to pay. The U.S. system on the other hand is in direct opposition to the utilitarian belief because access to the societal good of health care is only available to those who have the monetary resources or belong to a very specific group, not according to need.

Kantian theory tells people they ought to treat others as they want to be treated themselves. Furthermore, people should never be treated as a means to an end. In other words, don't use people for your own benefit. This holds true for individuals, corporations, and governments. Research provides a good example of this theory of justice. Research using human subjects should be done in such a way as to protect the subjects from treatment that would not be acceptable to you. This is reflected in the codes of ethics for research (Beauchamp and Childress 2012).

John Rawls and the Theory of Justice

One of the most influential philosophers in the field of health care and the just distribution of societal goods such as health care was John Rawls. His landmark book, *A Theory of Justice*, was published in 1971. His *justice as fairness* concept has been the basis of policy on a large-scale societal level in such diverse areas as economics, education, and health care ever since. Prior to this work, much of the discussion on health care ethics was centered on the individual patient/ provider interaction, not what the government or society as a whole should or should not do.

This theory of justice works so well because it includes basic concepts of social justice, utilitarianism, Kantian theory, and rights theories in one elegant theory. Rawls's theory is based on two principles that then guide moral decision making for society, governments, and individuals when it comes to dividing societal goods such as liberty, opportunity, income, wealth, and the basis of self-respect. The theory also addresses the differences in the natural benefits one is born with, but in no way deserved like health, intelligence, imagination, and position in society at birth. Health care, because of its special place in people's lives, includes and is influenced by all these goods. The first principle states that each person is to have an equal right to basic liberties compatible with a similar system of liberty for all. In other words, no one has more rights than one's neighbor; if one can have health care, all should. The second principle states that given that there are natural and social inequalities, they have to be handled so that they both give the least advantaged as much benefit as is possible. The theory would allow millions to be spent developing a new knee for a basketball star if and only if there were a way to give that same type of knee to a poor child with a congenital defect (a least advantaged person). Rawls further states that all societal benefits must be open to all under the fair equality of opportunity clause. This is the rationale for access to medical school or other public higher education regardless of gender, ethnic background, or other differences for all (Rawls 1971).

As we have seen in the ongoing health care reform debates and legal challenges to the Affordable Care Act, the delivery of health care services is special because it:

- Has the overarching goal of reducing pain and suffering
- Increases the quality of people's lives by prevention of disease and enhancing wellness and fitness
- Influences the opportunities a person has in society
- Has a historical, religious, and moral connotation
- Is unpredictable and intermittent in its need; it is not usually a continuous lifelong need, like food or shelter that is not affected by class or position

This last category of unpredictability is important in a theory of justice trying to account for a large population. There are of course diseases or risks that are greater and that occur more often in one class or position than another. It is, for instance, unlikely that a wealthy person, who was mentally sound, would be the victim of chronic starvation, nor is it likely that a person from the poverty zone in the United States would be made ill by improperly canned French escargot or Russian caviar. However, anyone from any class may develop cancer or pneumonia. These special features of health care complicate any discussion of the delivery system and justice. John Rawls's theory takes into account the need for both equal opportunity, the natural lottery of abilities and talents, the need for a Kantian test of respect for others, and our innate sense that justice and fairness should be the basis for something as important as health care. Under the Rawls theory of justice in health care, it would not be permissible to deny life and opportunity giving health benefits because someone was a person of color, poor, a woman or child, or any other special category, unless that benefit was not available to anyone else.

Women and Health Care Justice

The principles of John Rawls can be used to evaluate the health care system in the United States. In this example of using a moral theory to determine whether a system is fair or just, the case of women and the health care system will be examined. To understand how women are treated in the U.S. health care system, it is necessary to review the model of distribution of health care. In the United States, we have a market model of distribution, perhaps not a perfect model, but it comes closest to describing the system. From a Rawlsian perspective, if health care cannot be distributed in a way that satisfies the two principles of justice, the distribution method is unjust and should be changed.

Looking at women most easily makes the case for health care reform using a theory of justice. Health care distribution in the United States accounts for about 18 percent of its gross domestic product, or over $8,000 per person (http://www.oecd.org/infobycountry).

Yet women, who make up over 50 percent of the population, do not enjoy 50 percent of its benefits (National Women's Law Center 2004). Because women do not enjoy equal access to the opportunities of employment in the health care field (fewer women than men are high-paying providers, administrators, or researchers), they are disadvantaged. They also do not have the financial resources (the median income of women is still less by far than that for men) to compete with males for access to service, access to the benefits of research or treatments. Because a market model distributes health care in the United States by exchanging the benefits of health care for a monetary exchange and women are at an economic disadvantage, women qualify under the theory of justice as least advantaged. The plight of women of color is even more dismal.

Women interact with the health care system at critical points in their lives: when giving birth, at menopause, and in old age. Yet, they are disadvantaged even at these points. A woman having a baby in the United States in 2014 had less chance of her child living than if she has had the baby in Cuba, which has a universal health care system (www.cia.gov/library/publications/the-world-factbook/rankorder/2091rank.html). As she reached menopause in the last four decades, she was given drugs that were known to be dangerous. For example, although the drug manufacturers and the FDA knew of the dangers connected to estrogen use, that information was withheld from women from the first studies indicating serious problems in the 1980s to the first black box warning in 2002 for further testing by drug companies (Hulley 2004). But when the drug was used for men for prostate cancer, a very specific warning about its dangers was included (www.ourbodiesourselves.org). This is clearly a case of unequal treatment based on gender and unacceptable under any theory of justice.

Women's issues in old age have very low research priority because they are primarily chronic conditions like heart failure and arthritis. In fact, private foundations are now doing most of the research into breast cancer and arthritis, sponsored mostly by women themselves. However, there is a great deal of government-funded research into disease and conditions of men such as acute heart conditions, prostate cancer, and replacements of knees and hips. Women are consistently treated with disrespect by the health providers and have last place on claims for research money to decrease their morbidity. In addition, the mortality of both mother and infants in the United States is extremely high for an industrialized country—13th in the world. This is not what one would have expected from a just health care system. Indeed, using the Rawlsian theory, it is obvious that the market model of health care is not a just distribution system. It is this conclusion that fuels the continuing call for meaningful health care reform in the United States.

Using the Rawlsian theory to evaluate other countries is a good way to compare the justice and fairness of systems. The Swedish system, for example, is a wholly nationalized system. Medical, dental, and pharmaceutical needs are met for all citizens by government-sponsored agencies. The basic thrust of the system is to keep people well. As a result, the Swedish people enjoy some of the best health care in the world, their life expectancy is one of the highest (81 years), and the maternal and infant mortality is the lowest in the world. In addition, they spend only about one-half the money per person ($4,000) on health care as does the United States ($8,000). However, the marginal personal income tax in Sweden is over 50 percent, one of the highest rates in the world. The Swedish health system does not allow unequal treatment on the basis of wealth or income shares. From a Rawlsian perspective, the Swedish health system has several promising features: universal access and equity of care, participation by the public in the allocation of health resources process, regulation of the private sector to ensure against vast income disparities, and a philosophy that emphasizes wellness and the dignity of the person. Rawlsian principles would judge it to be more just than the U.S. system on the basis of equity of resource allocation treatment of those who by their health needs would be classed as least advantaged.

This same critique and conclusion could be done with any of the other countries that have health care systems that ensure universal access and care for all citizens that need it. The countries that meet the test of justice and fairness for their health care systems would include Great Britain, France, Germany, Japan, and Canada to name a few (www.oecd.org/infobycountry).

Career Profile: Social Scientists and Patient Advocates

How do we learn about cultures such as the Pima Indians or the Hmong or even the subcultures of our own community? Social scientists such as sociologists and anthropologists provide much of the research that informs public policy decisions. Sociology is the study of social relationships and institutions. Anthropology is the study of past and present humans. Both fields have multiple subspecialties. Courses in these fields are often included in the requirements for health care professions because they expand the awareness and cultural competency of practitioners. Students who obtain a bachelor's degree in sociology or anthropology work in a wide range of career fields. Those who wish to conduct research generally obtain a master's degree and doctorate and then work for colleges and universities, government agencies, and community organizations.

In addition to cultural competency, the field of health care is increasingly concerned about rights and ethics. You've seen throughout this text that different professions are bound by their respective codes of ethics. You've explored certain philosophical approaches to the big dilemmas in health care. This protective concern has created a new career—the patient advocate. Support, education, and clinical liaison are the three areas of responsibility, although the specifics depend on the patient's needs. In the support role, the advocate might help a family obtain financial assistance or choose an insurance plan or purchase health care materials. The advocate can usually connect the patient with a network of contacts that assist in all parts of process. In the education role, the advocate might help the patient and her family learn how to live with dietary restrictions or long-term effects of a disease. In the role of clinical liaison, the advocate may be present at appointments with the health care provider or work with the patient's employer. The advocate clearly needs a high level of understanding of the systems the patient encounters, as well as the ability to maintain patient privacy. Currently there are no educational or licensing requirements to become an advocate, although there are a few colleges that are offering courses and short-term programs. The fees charged by the advocate vary considerably depending on the experience and training of the advocate and the nature of the services being provided. The Alliance of Professional Health Advocates is a membership organization for private, professional advocates. The National Patient Advocate Foundation is a U.S. not-for-profit organization that focuses on regulatory and legislative reform.

Summary

Culture refers to integrated patterns of human behavior that include the language, thoughts, communications, actions, customs, beliefs, values, and institutions of racial, ethnic, religious, gender, age, or social groups. Competence implies having the capacity to function effectively as an individual and an organization within the context of the cultural beliefs, behaviors, and needs presented by consumers and their communities.

Cultural competence is the ability of health organizations and practitioners to recognize the cultural beliefs, values, attitudes, traditions, language preferences, and health practices of specific cultural groups and to apply that knowledge to produce positive health outcomes. Competency includes communicating in a manner that is linguistically and culturally appropriate.

Health literacy is the ability of the individual to understand health care providers' information such as prescription instructions, disease brochures, and health care instructions. Researchers have developed tools for the health professional to use in assessing health literacy and providing linguistically appropriate patient education materials. Health literacy improves health outcomes.

Health care ethics addresses large concepts such as respect for autonomy, nonmaleficence (do no harm), beneficence (do good), justice, veracity (truth telling), privacy, confidentiality, and professional roles. Health care ethics also provides health care professionals with their codes of ethics. These codes demand a certain standard of behavior if one is to be in good standing with the health care professions. There are universal principles including veracity (telling the truth) and confidentiality that are the cornerstones of professional behavior and duty to patients. Along with the virtues of compassion, integrity, trustworthiness, and wisdom, these principles guide the health care professional in the care of patients. There are several major ethical theories used to help health policy makers and governments divide the pie. The theory of John Rawls includes basic concepts of social justice, utilitarianism, Kantian, and rights theories. It examines the market model of health care distribution to determine the justice and fairness of our health care system.

Questions for Review

1. What is cultural competency?
2. Why is cultural competency important?
3. Describe health literacy.
4. How is it different from regular literacy and the ability to read?
5. How is health literacy assessed?
6. Define the major health ethics principles.
7. What are the advantages of John Rawls's theory of justice?
8. What are the principles and virtues of professionalism?

Questions for Discussion

1. Refer to the chapter profile. Why was cultural competency and health literacy so important for health care providers in caring for the Pima Indians?
2. Who should be trained in cultural competency and health literacy?
3. How many cultures are represented by the students in your classroom today? Discuss the different health care traditions represented by those cultures.
4. Is cultural competency an ethical question, and why?

5. Discuss health care reform in terms of ethical theories.
6. Describe a societal ethical dilemma and then apply two different principles of ethics to it and defend your decision in terms of that principle.
7. How do the cultural aspects listed in Table 13.2 impact health care, giving specific examples?

Chapter References

Beauchamp, T. L., and J. F. Childress. 2012. *Principles of biomedical ethics*. 7th ed. New York, NY and Oxford, England: Oxford University Press.

www.cdc.gov/diabetes/pubs/statsreport14/national-diabetes-report-web.pdf.

Center for Linguistic and Cultural Competency in Health Care, Office of Minority Health (www. minorityhealth.hhs.gov).

www.cia.gov/library/publications/the-world-factbook/rankorder/2091rank.html.

Culture and Ethnicity in Medicine—Bioethics Resources on the Web—National Institutes of Health (http://bioethics.od.nih.gov/culturalcomp.html).

Fadiman, A. 1997. *The spirit catches you and you fall down: A Hmong girl, her American doctors, and the collision of two cultures*. New York: Farrar, Straus, and Giroux.

Henslin, J. M. 2014. *Sociology: A down-to-earth approach*. 12th ed. Upper Saddle River, NJ: Prentice Hall.

Hulley, S. 2004. The WHI Estrogen-Alone Trial—Do things look any better? *JAMA* 291: 1769–1771.

Indian Health Service Communication Tool Kit (www.ihs.gov/healthcommunications/index.cfm?module=dsp_hc_toolkit).

Indian Health Service: White paper on Health Literacy#15A646 – accessed 5/09/2010 (www.ihs.gov/healthcommunications).

National Center for Cultural Competence, Georgetown University (www11.georgetown.edu/research/gucchd/nccc/foundations/frameworks).

National diabetes statistics 2007 (http://diabetes.niddk.nih.gov/dm/pubs/statistics/).

National Institute of Diabetes and Digestive and Kidney Diseases (NIDDK) (www.diabetes.niddk.nih.gov/DM/pubs/pima).

National Women's Law Center and the Oregon Health & Science University. 2004. *Making the grade on women's health: A national and state-by-state report card*. Washington, DC: Author.

Organization for Employment, Labour & Social Affairs, OECD Health Data 2009 (www. oecd.org/infobycountry).

Our Bodies Ourselves (www.ourbodiesourselves.org/book/menoexcertp.asp?id=58&chaptered=31).

Rawls, J. 1971. *A theory of justice*. Cambridge, MA: Harvard University Press.

UNICEF (www.unicef.org/infobycountry/cuba).

UNICEF (www.unicef.org/infobycountry/usa).

Women's Health Initiative. (www.nhlhi.nih.gov/whi/e-a_advisory.htm).

For Additional Information

Bioethics Resources on the Web http://bioethics.od.nih.gov.

Coughlin, S. *Ethical issues in epidemiologic research and public health practice*. Atlanta, GA: Epidemiology and Applied Research Branch, Division of Cancer Prevention and Control, National Center for Chronic Disease Prevention and Health Promotion, Centers for Disease Control and Prevention. Available at www.ete-online.com/content/3/1/16.

Drugwatch (www.drugwatch.com/premarian).

Health Care: The White House (www.whitehouse.gov/issues/health-care).

HealthReform.gov (www.healthreform.gov/).

Hoyert, D. L. 2007. Maternal mortality and related concepts. National Center for Health Statistics. *Vital Health Statistics* 3(33).

Obasogie, O., and D. Winickoff. 2006. *When is the racial pharmacy bad medicine?* Available at www.thehastingscenter.org/Bioethicsforum/.

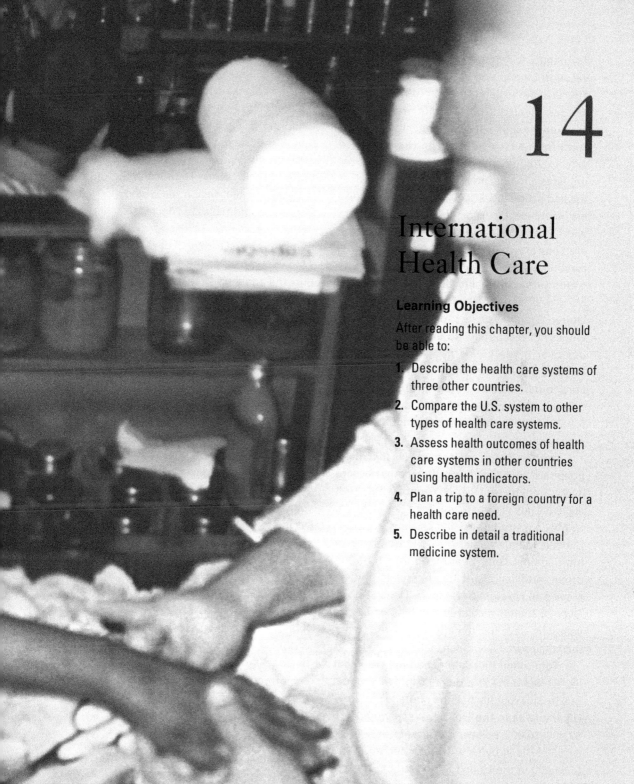

14

International Health Care

Learning Objectives

After reading this chapter, you should be able to:

1. Describe the health care systems of three other countries.
2. Compare the U.S. system to other types of health care systems.
3. Assess health outcomes of health care systems in other countries using health indicators.
4. Plan a trip to a foreign country for a health care need.
5. Describe in detail a traditional medicine system.

Dental Vacation in Mexico

Tom and Becky returned from their Mexican vacation tanned and with wonderful smiles. This was particularly true for Tom. Before he left for Mexico, Tom's smile was literally crooked because he was missing several teeth from a bicycle accident. His insurance was inadequate to cover the expense of implants, crowns, and bridges. The U.S. dentist had estimated $12,000 above and beyond his insurance. Like most dental policies, there was a yearly cap on expenses that barely covered one crown, let alone a whole mouth restoration. Tom had heard from a friend that he could get good quality dental work done in Mexico for about half what it would be in the United States. Tom's job involved a lot of work with the public, so stringing the work out over 4 years was not a viable option. He and Becky started researching dental care outside the United States. Friends thought they were crazy: after all, wasn't all foreign health care dangerous and prone to complications?

The first thing Tom learned was that many hospitals and clinics in other countries are accredited by the same organization that accredits hospitals here, the Joint Commission. In Mexico, the largest health care provider, Christus Muguerza, has the Joint Commission International Gold Seal of Approval among other certifications. It has hospitals both in Mexico and in eight states in the United States. Over 28 countries cater to a million patients a year who have health care in a country other than their own (Woodman 2007).

Tom found he could get all the work that he needed done in a dental clinic in Tijuana, Mexico, for roughly half the quoted U.S. price. His implants in the United States would run $2,400–$3,000 apiece; in Tijuana, they were $1,500. His crowns were quoted as $800 to $1,000 in the United States, and in Mexico $375. He could go to Mexico to have his dental work done, take Becky and stay in a four star hotel for 2 weeks, and still save about $3,000. Tom and Becky took the Amtrak train from their home in Portland, Oregon, to San Diego, California, hopped a shuttle from the train station to the border, and the resort shuttle met them on the other side of the border and took them to their resort. The next day, Tom met with the dentist, taking his X-rays and other information from his U.S. dentist with him. The dentist examined Tom and made appointments for the next several days to do the work. Tom reported that the thing that impressed him the most at first was the fact that the dentist gave him his full attention at each appointment—no going from room to room, working on several people at once. He made the crowns himself, fitting them to Tom at each stage, so no need for a long wait between stages. The resort was geared for the medical traveler and provided transportation from the resort to the clinic each day and special foods and had a pharmacy on site. The dentist gave Tom his cell phone number with instructions to call him if there were any problems. The work was completed with no complications. In Tom's mind, this was the best dental experience of his life.

More and more countries are becoming medical tourism destinations. Medical tourism statistics revealed an anticipated growth of the industry from about $40 billion in 2004 to $100 billion by 2012. It was also estimated that a million and a half Americans sought health care outside the United States in 2008. So, pack your bags for a face-lift in Rio de Janeiro, a tummy tuck in Costa Rica, or a hip replacement in Canada.

Sources: Woodman, J. 2007. *Patients beyond borders*. Chapel Hill, NC: Healthy Travel Media: Joint Commission (http://www.medicaltravel.com.mx/certifications); http://www.understanding-medicaltourism.com/medical-tourism-statistics.php.

Introduction

We live in a global community and that community includes health care. This book has up to this point given you a look at the major segments of the U.S. system. This chapter will give an overview of some of the global systems. Although all countries have a health care system of some sort, we have chosen only a few to examine. To compare countries and how well their health care system works, health indicators such as life expectancy, spending on health care, infant and maternal mortality, and the percentage of the citizens covered by the system are used by scientists, researchers, and policy makers.

Both Canada and Mexico are our neighbors, and people travel with relative ease to both countries for business, pleasure, and health care. So, we will explore both those systems. The British system is the oldest national health care system and a model for many other countries and will be reviewed here. The French and German systems are well-established systems with both strong public and private segments. India is without a doubt the largest system, with a strong traditional medicine and homeopathic system as well as a flourishing Western-style component.

Data about these systems are presented in Table 14.1. Keep in mind our own system as you review the global perspective. When compared to other developed countries such as the United Kingdom, Canada, France, or Japan, the United States spends more on health per capita, yet has poorer outcomes on measures such as infant and maternal mortality rates. Despite improvements in reducing the number of uninsured due to the Affordable Care Act, the percentage of citizens covered in the United States lags behind those of other countries.

Health Care Delivery Systems

The most common system for delivering health care around the globe is what is called a **Single-Payer system**. A single-payer system is the financing of the costs of delivering universal health care for an entire population through a single insurance pool out of which costs are paid. This is the system those countries with universal access and treatment for all citizens use. All the health care costs are billed to and paid by a single agency within the country, state, or province. Health care providers do not usually bill individual services under this plan, but bill the cost of running the clinic, hospital, or home health unit directly to the government. This system is used in all the Scandinavian countries, Canada, Australia, New Zealand, the United Kingdom, Taiwan, Cuba, and a variation of it in France, Germany, Spain, Italy, and other countries with universal health care as a societal benefit.

Single-Payer system
The financing of the costs of delivering health care for an entire population through a single insurance pool out of which costs are met. Canada and the United Kingdom are good examples.

The United States and a handful of developing countries use the market economy model to deliver health care. As described in Chapter 2, in a market economy model system, the price and distribution of goods, in this case health care, is determined by supply and demand. It allows the price of health care to increase as demand increases and tends to concentrate service in areas of high population regardless of the need of more rural areas. In addition, if the disease or condition does not generate enough demand, there is little incentive to treat or research the

Table 14.1 *International Comparison of Selected Health Indicators and Spending*

	United States	United Kingdom	Mexico	Canada	Germany	France	Japan	India
System	Market <65 Single payer >65 Universal veterans	Universal Single payer	3% Market 97% public/ universal	Universal/ Private	Universal Insurance Mandated Private insurance	Universal coverage	Universal coverage	Private Traditional government
Population in millions	313.9	63.7	117.1	34	81.9	63.5	127.5	1,236.7 billion
Life expectancy	80.2	81.0	74.4	81.5	81.0	80.9	83.2	63.7
HC spending as part of GDP	16.9%	9.3%	10.9%	9.8%	11.3%	11.6%	10.3%	5.2%
Per person spending	$8,475	$3,011	$877	$4,045	$3,995	$3,476	$3,222	NA
Infant mortality/ 1,000 births	5.96	4.1	13.3	4.8	3.3	3.5	2.2	49.8
Maternal mortality/ 100,000 live births	28	8	49	11	7	9	6	190
Percentage of citizens covered	87%	100%	100%	100%	100%	100%	100%	NA

Sources: https://data.oecd.org/pop/population.htm; www.compareyourcountry.org/health?cr=oecd&cr1=oecd&lg=en&page=2#; www.oecd.org/els/family/CO1_1_Infant%20mortality_updated1May2014.pdf; www.oecd.org/health/health-systems/Table-of-Content-Metadata-OECD-Health-Statistics-2014.pdf; www.who.int/reproductivehealth/publications/monitoring/maternal-mortality-2013/en/ Table 2. Trends in estimates of maternal mortality ratio (MMR, maternal deaths per 100,000 live births), 1990–2013, by country, WHO.Int; www.cdc.gov/nchs/fastats/infant-health.htm.

condition. Many countries like Japan use a mixed model in which there is mandatory insurance, and the delivery model is a private market model. The market model of health care delivery treats health care like any other product or service, ignoring the very special aspects of health care described in Chapter 13. Generally, we do not choose to have a stroke or break a leg, so there is no freedom of choice involved in our spending of resources. This would seem to invalidate the market model as a sustainable delivery system. Costs rise very rapidly in this system, and there is great disparity between levels of providers with some physicians earning many millions of dollars a year, while nurses and other providers earn a small fraction of that as described in the chapters on health care providers.

The differences in the models of health care delivery are studied by looking at the efficiency and outcomes of the system. We will examine a few next. The U.S. system is not included in this chapter as it has been extensively examined in the previous chapters.

Mexico

Public institutions, state and federal governments, private providers, and private hospitals and clinics provide health care in Mexico. Mexico was in the world spotlight in 2009 during the outbreak of the pandemic H1N1 flu outbreak.

History

The first hospital in Mexico was founded in 1791 by the Bishop of Guadalajara, the Hospicio Cabanas. It is not only a functioning hospital today, but is the largest health complex in Central and Latin America and is a World Heritage site. The Mexican Social Security Institute, IMSS (Instituto Mexicano del Seguro Social), was founded in 1943 to provide public health care to all Mexican citizens. In 2003, the Mexican government launched a universal health care plan.

Mexican Health Care Delivery System

The system in Mexico is a three-part system (private, public, and universal) with different levels of care, provider payment, and delivery options depending on the employment status and income of the citizen.

The private system covers roughly 3 percent of the population and caters to the wealthy of the country and the booming medical tourism trade. It is a combination of private insurers who facilitate access to state of the art and very high-quality health care and people who are covered by the public system but pay out of pocket for higher-quality services. Non-Mexicans can purchase health care in Mexico by private insurers—both Mexican and American, out-of-pocket payments and other governments' national plans (British, Canadian, and French), who reimburse Mexico for their citizens' care. Private-sector health care is booming in Mexico, partly due to medical tourism. U.S. citizens like Tom flock to Mexico for dental work, cosmetic surgery, cardiac procedures, orthopedic procedures, and ophthalmology procedures. Mexico is also a popular retirement destination for U.S. and Canadian citizens, further increasing the demand for high-quality care. Many Mexican physicians are trained in the United States, and increasingly U.S. physicians are trained in Mexico.

The public system in Mexico covers wage earners, state employees, and the military. An estimated 50 million workers pay into an insurance plan according to their wages. The IMSS or Mexican Social Security System operates its own clinics and hospitals for insured workers. The quality of these state-run clinics and hospitals varies a good deal. Workers may also opt to use the private system and pay the out-of-pocket expenses. Some 17 million state employees pay into a separate plan administered through the Institute of Security and Social Services, which runs its own clinics and hospitals. The military and employees of the state-owned petroleum company, Pemex, are covered through their own insurance programs. The remaining uninsured Mexicans—about 40 percent of the population—fall under the umbrella of the universal health care plan known as the Popular Health Insurance plan. It was initiated in 2003 with the goal of reducing health care inequities and serving the poorest of citizens. Families pay a premium to join dependent on income (about 20 percent of families pay no premiums) and are required to visit clinics for preventive care (http://content.healthaffairs.org/cgi/content/full/24/6/1467).

Statistics

Universal health in Mexico is credited with an increase in positive health care outcomes in Mexico and reducing catastrophic health cost by as much as 9 percent (*Lancet* 2012). Mexican children now receive the same vaccinations as Canadian children. Malaria and TB cases have dropped. Per capita spending in Mexico for health care is about half of what is spent in the United States.

Canada

The Canadian system for health care delivery can be described as a mixed system because it is possible to have completely private health care with the patient paying the provider. However, most Canadian health care is provided through the single-payer model. Each province in Canada has the constitutional option to opt out of this system, although none have to date. All physician, hospital, pharmaceutical, and clinic fees are set and paid for by the government. A health care provider cannot charge more than the government fee, even if the patient is not covered by the public system or is from another country, unless the provider opts out of the system altogether. Other health care expenses such as dentistry and optometry are wholly private-sector operations. Each person who enrolls in the program is given a health care card, much like the Medicare card in the United States. All people have the same plan (http://www.hc-sc.gc.ca).

In recent years, American citizens have increasingly gone to Canada to purchase prescription drugs and be treated for certain illnesses. U.S. citizens take advantage of the high quality and lower cost of Canadian health care. Canadians also come to the United States for elective surgeries such as hip and heart. Canadians travel to the United States for health care for specialized procedures not available in Canada and in some cases to avoid long waiting times.

History

The early French settlers founded Catholic hospitals in the 1800s. Health care in Canada was private until 1946. At that time, the province of Saskatchewan introduced universal health care coverage. Over the next 10 years, the remaining nine provinces introduced similar coverage. In 1957, the Hospital and Diagnostic Services Act was passed through which the federal government paid 50 percent of costs of the health care programs in all 10 provinces. In 1966, the Medical Care Act was passed that instituted the universal coverage countrywide. The Canada Health Act was passed in 1984 that prohibited extra user fees and extra physician billing fees. The Canadian system, which blends universal health coverage with private-sector fee-for-service, is often seen as a model for U.S. health care reform in current and future discussions.

Delivery

The majority of health care in Canada (75%) is funded publicly and delivered privately. The private-sector spending is about 30 percent of the total, primarily for services not covered by Canadian Medicare such as dentistry, optometry, some prescription drugs, cosmetic surgery, and for, in some provinces, priority access to health care services. Canadians may also purchase supplementary private health insurance for these services; about 65 percent of the population has this coverage.

The actual delivery of services is the responsibility of the provinces and territories. Although privately funded, most of the services are provided by private enterprises. Most physicians do not receive a salary, but are paid on a fee-for-service basis. They in turn pay their staff, much like private practice physicians in the United States. The role of the federal government is to:

- Provide the funds to deliver the services to the provinces
- Set and administer the principles of the national health care system
- Deliver services to specific special groups—veterans, First Nation Peoples, and the Inuit people
- Provide public health, health protection programs, and health care research

Both Canadian citizens and health care providers report high approval ratings for this system (Health Canada http://www.hc-sc.gc.ca).

Statistics

In 2012, Canada spent 9.8 percent of GDP on health care, or U.S. $4,045 per capita. Of that, approximately 70 percent was government expenditure, according to the World Health Organization (WHO) (Canada http://www.who.int/countries/can).

India

India has a population of over 1 billion people, with only seven physicians per 10,000 people, according to WHO. India has no central health care system, unlike the other countries we have reviewed. The responsibility for health care is through a system of primary care centers, traditional medicine practitioners, and hospitals. The rural health care system treats less complicated cases and then funnels difficult cases to the urban centers. The system is divided between the modern Western style health care and the traditional systems and homeopathy. Traditional medicine has been practiced in India for thousands of years. Traditional systems include Ayurveda, Unani, Siddha, Yoga, naturopathy, and homeopathy. These are major delivery systems in India; they treat more people than the modern Western-style clinics and hospitals. There are 3,204 traditional hospitals and 725,000 practitioners in India, according to the Ministry of Health (http://www.india.gov.in/citizen/health/health.php).

India is also a major medical tourism destination for Western-style procedures. India hosts several million foreign visitors seeking high-quality, low-cost health care. Because foreigners pay directly, this form of tourism pumps billions into the Indian economy. Cardiovascular procedures top the list (http://www.indianhealthcare.in).

Ayurvedic Medicine—Up Close

Traditional medicine has long been an interest of this author. In 2014 I was given a unique chance to study one of the world's oldest systems up close and personal. I spent a month at an Ayurvedic Clinic in Sri Lanka, a small island nation off the coast of India that, with India, is a major user of this system of health care. The clinic housed a World Health Organization Medicinal Plant Repository, which gave me an opportunity to observe the herb-based system from growing to dispensing.

The Ayurvedic system is built on the balance in the body of three elements: Vata, Pitta, and Kapha. Health or illness depends on the presence or absence of a balanced state. The diagnosis takes into consideration not only the person's physical state, but also the mental condition, and the person's position in society. The system is the very definition of holistic. The treatments include diet, massage and other bodywork, spiritual guidance, and medicines. People come from all over the world to be treated here by the traditional medicine practitioners.

I followed the process of patient admission, treatment, and follow-up by becoming a patient myself and collaborating with the Ayurvedic physicians to better understand this complex system and its impact on the population of several countries—India, Sri Lanka, and Myanmar. Allopathic (Western) medicine is practiced side by side with the traditional system; patients often have both an allopathic and Ayurvedic practitioner. In my case all my Ayurvedic physicians and pharmacists had had training in a Western system as well as the traditional.

The consultation started as any medical exam would with physical measurements of height, weight, BP, temperature, respirations, heart rate, and lab work, the standard chemistry screen—all done by the physician herself. After this she did an extensive history of illness, medications, surgery, allergies, daily habits, psychological status, and a different type of physical exam which included her just looking at me and asking me to show my tongue, cross eyes, and some muscle tone demonstrations. After this 30-page/1-hour-long exam, she prescribed a regimen of diet, exercise (yoga and Tai Chi), massage, herbal wraps, herbal baths, acupuncture, and plant-based medicines. I was taken off all Western drugs for the month. When I returned to the United States, my regular physician discontinued some entirely, and others had the dosage reduced by half or three-quarters.

My Ayurvedic physician set goals for my blood pressure, weight, and flexibility. The daily routine was somewhat rigorous. I started the day at 6 A.M. with 90 minutes of yoga, followed by a swim in either the pool or ocean. Then I had breakfast (also a prescription), acupuncture, massage, herbal wrap, herbal bath, lunch, rest, leisure activity of my choice, 5 P.M. Tai Chi, dinner, and a cultural activity. In the Ayurvedic tradition, diet, socialization, and food for the mind are as important as the medications. Every day I had decoctions to take both as pill form and as drinks with meals. As you might guess, there was no caffeine, meat, or alcohol; very little dairy; no refined sugar; and very little fat in the diet. Not any wonder I dropped weight and have kept it off, lowered my blood pressure and cholesterol (all which have remained low), and could get into yoga positions I had not dreamed possible by the end of the month. Of course, this was a very intensive program designed for the drop-in Westerner.

The population of Sri Lanka is primarily Hindu or Buddhist, so meat, caffeine, and alcohol are not common. Ayurvedic practitioners deliver about 80 percent of the medical care in Sri Lanka. The government sponsors Ayurvedic hospitals and clinics. It is a regular part of the health care system. If you have the flu or break a bone, the first recourse is this traditional medicine model. Because this is the oldest medical system in the world with texts dating back to 600 BCE and oral traditions dating back 8,000 years, they are pretty good at the day-to-day business of health care. There are eight specialties in this system: internal medicine; surgery; eyes, ears, nose, and throat; pediatrics including obstetrics and gynecology; psychology and psychiatry; toxicology; nutrition and prevention and promotion of health; and sexual function.

The infrastructure of the Sri Lankan health system was dealt a severe blow by the tsunami in 2004, with 17 hospitals destroyed or heavily damaged, 35,000 lives lost, over 100,000 people displaced, and the disappearance of whole villages. The country is slowly recovering from this tragedy, but the scars remain. The clinic I resided in had been severely damaged and several buildings demolished; the water line is still visible in the pharmacy and several buildings. Thousands of people died along this stretch of the coast. I was there for the tenth anniversary of the disaster and heard firsthand many stories of people doing heroic things to save others.

Health Outcomes

Sri Lanka spends 2 percent of its GDP on health care and has a maternal mortality rate of 28/100,000, whereas the United States spends 17.9 percent of its GDP and has a maternal mortality rate of 29/100,000. From these statistics, it appears that the dual traditional medicine/allopathic system of Sri Lanka is a very cost-effective system. The delivery of traditional medicine is much cheaper than that of Western systems. More people can be served, with less expense and have outcomes that surpass or equal the allopathic system of the United States.

The system is known in the United States. Walk into any major U.S. grocery store, and you will find Ayurvedic teas and herbs in the health foods section. Deepak Chopra popularized Ayurvedic medicine in the United States, although it has been popular in Europe since the 1800s as Europeans colonized and traded with both India and Sri Lanka. In fact, a Portuguese family founded the clinic I attended. This system is a very good example of the types of traditional medicine found around the world: in Asia, Africa, South America, Native American Indians, and Island Nations like Australia and New Zealand. Although allopathic medicine replaces knees and implants bionic sensory enhancers, traditional medicine treats the day-to-day illnesses and promotes healthy people for a fraction of the cost. Those countries that blend the two seamlessly appear to have the best of both worlds.

Sources: www.commonwealthhealth.org/asia/sri_lanka/child_and_maternal_health_in_sri_lanka/; www.commonwealthhealth.org/asia/sri_lanka/

Summary

Health care in a global community ranges from single-payer systems to traditional medicine systems. Very few systems look like our own system, but our system has aspects of most of the other systems embedded in it. Medical tourism in the past was to a large extent an American experience with people from all over the world coming here for advanced procedures and care. That trend is reversing because of the high cost of American health care and the increasing sophistication of other health care systems. People are going to all corners of the globe for health care from prescription medicines in Canada to heart surgery in India.

To compare countries and how well their health care system works, health indicators such as life expectancy, spending on health care, infant and maternal mortality, and the percentage of the citizens covered by the system are used.

Questions for Review

1. What is a single-payer system?
2. Name two countries with single-payer systems.
3. Compare and contrast the U.S. system with a single-payer system.
4. Describe the Canadian health care system.
5. Describe a traditional health care system.
6. Which country spends the most/least on health care?
7. In which country is the risk of dying during childbirth the lowest/highest?
8. In which country do children under the age of one die the most/least?
9. In which country do people live the longest/shortest?
10. What is medical tourism?

Questions for Discussion

1. What type of health care system would you like to live under?
2. Is health care better in the United States? Why or why not? What indicators did you use to define "better"?
3. Should basic indicators of health care be the only measure of a system's success? What other indicators would you use?
4. Would you travel to a foreign country as Tom (see the chapter profile) did for health care to save money?

Chapter References

www.cdc.gov/nchs/fastats/infant-health.htm
www.commonwealthhealth.org/asia/sri_lanka/child_and_maternal_health_in_sri_lanka
www.commonwealthhealth.org/asia/sri_lanka/
www.compareyourcountry.org/health?cr=oecd&cr1=oecd&lg=en&page=2#
https://data.oecd.org/pop/population.htm
Department of Health—England (http://www.dh.gov.uk).
Health Canada (http://www.hc-sc.gc.ca).
India Brand Equity Foundation (http://www.ibef.org).
Indian Citizen Health (http://www.india.gov.in/citizen/health/health.php).
Indian Health Care (http://www.indianhealthcare.in).

Joint Commission (http://www.medicaltravel.com.mx/certifications).

The Lancet. 2012. Mexico: Celebrating universal health coverage. Vol. 380, No. 9842, p. 622, 18 August 2012.

National Health Service—England (http://www.nhs.uk).

www.oecd.org/els/family/CO1_1_Infant%20mortality_updated1May2014.pdf

www.oecd.org/health/health-systems/Table-of-Content-Metadata-OECD-Health-Statistics-2014.pdf

Organization for Employment, Labour and Social Affairs (http://www.oecd.org/health/healthataglance).

Understanding Medical Tourism (http://www.understanding-medicaltourism.com/medical-tourism-statistics.php).

UNESCO—World Heritage site—Hospicio Cabanas (http://whc.unesco.org/archive/advisory_body_evaluation/815.pdf).

UNICEF (http://www.unicef.org/infobycountry/).

UNICEF—Mexico (http://www.unicef.org/infobycountry/mexico_statistics.html).

Woodman, J. 2007. *Patients beyond borders.* Chapel Hill, NC: Healthy Travel Media.

www.who.int/reproductivehealth/publications/monitoring/maternal-mortality-2013/en/ Table 2. Trends in estimates of maternal mortality ratio (MMR, maternal deaths per 100,000 live births), 1990–2013, by country, WHO.Int.

World Health Organization (http://apps.who.int/whosis/database).

World Health Organization Canada (http://www.who.int/countries/can).

For Additional Information

Organization for Employment, Labour and Social Affairs (http://www.oecd.org/health/healthataglance).

Glossary

Accounting – The business function that tracks flows of payments into and out of a business.

Activities of daily living – Basic activities such as mobility, eating, toileting, dressing, and bathing.

Actuary – A professional who calculates insurance and annuity risks, premiums, and dividends.

Acute care – Short-term medical care provided to a patient with an immediate need for care.

ADN (associate degree in nursing) – An associate's program typically takes 2 years to complete and is usually offered by a community college.

Advanced practice nurse – A nurse who has obtained a master's degree in a clinical specialty.

Aging in place – A philosophy that allows the aging person or couple to stay in their living situation while growing older with increasing levels of personal and medical assistance as needed. These are adult living communities where the range is from individual homes to a skilled nursing facility in one complex.

Allopathic medicine – A process of treating disease by using standard treatments, such as surgery and drugs.

Alzheimer's disease – A degenerative disorder that affects the brain and causes dementia.

Ambulatory care – Medical care provided in an office setting to a mobile patient.

Antigenic drift – Describes the gradual and continuous changes in the genetic makeup of some viruses such as the Type B flu virus.

Antitrust law – An area of federal law which prohibits monopolization and other activities that lessen competition in the marketplace.

Assessment – The process of determining the health needs of a community.

Assisted living facilities (ALFs) – Homes or apartment-like living spaces that allow for independent activities such as cooking and bathing and also provide care such as medication or treatment delivery; a nonmedical model of chronic care living arrangements.

Assurance – The process of making sure that correct actions are taken to protect community health.

Benefits – The items that are covered under an insurance plan. Also referred to as coverage.

Biochemical – Involving chemical substances present in living organisms, such as dopamine.

Blind random trial – A clinical trial method in which no one knows which drugs the participants are receiving until the trial is finished.

Block grants – Money granted by the national government to a state government with few restrictions on its spending. This can be contrasted with a categorical grant, which has strict and specific provisions on the way it is to be spent.

Board certification – A physician may become board certified by completing additional years of residency in the specialty and passing an exam.

BSN (Bachelor of Science in Nursing) – A bachelor's program that usually takes 4 years to complete.

Burden of disease – The cost of a disease in terms of the individual, family, and community disability, including lost work, family relationships, and community participation.

Burnout – A psychological condition in which a person loses the ability to care and becomes apathetic. Stress and overwork are thought to cause burnout.

Business – The activity of providing goods and services to customers for profit.

Business cycle – Regular cycles of decline and growth in an economy over a time period.

Capitation – A payment method under which each patient is entitled to receive a set dollar amount of services in each time period.

Case – A term used in health statistics to refer to each person who has a disease.

Centers for Disease Control and Prevention (CDC) – A group of federal governmental agencies responsible for collecting and interpreting health care statistics.

249

Centers for Medicare & Medicaid Services (CMS) – The federal agency that administers the Medicare and Medicaid programs; previously known as the Health Care Financing Administration (HCFA).

Certified nurse-midwife (CNM) – An advanced practice nurse who provides prenatal and postpartum care and delivers infants.

Certified registered nurse anesthetist (CRNA) – An advanced practice nurse who specializes in anesthesia.

Children's Health Insurance Program (CHIP) – A federal program that targets low-income children whose parents do not qualify for Medicaid, yet are unable to afford private health insurance.

Chronic condition – An illness or injury lasting more than 90 days; a non-acute illness such as asthma.

Clinical nurse specialist (CNS) – An advanced practice nurse who specializes in a field such as oncology, neonatal care, or mental health.

Clinical trial – The process of testing a new drug, treatment, or medical device on humans in a controlled manner.

CME (Continuing Medical Education) – The state requirement that physicians receive a certain amount of additional training and education to remain licensed.

CNA (Certified Nursing Assistant) – A nurse's aide who has received the credential of CNA.

Cognitive – Relating to the process of thinking or acquiring knowledge. Cognitive diseases disrupt the ability to acquire or remember knowledge.

Communicable disease – A disease that spreads from person to person; another term for infectious disease.

Community hospital – Non-federal hospital facilities available to the public.

Compliance program – A program that is implemented in a business to ensure that it stays in compliance with current legislation, especially changes in the Medicare or Medicaid programs.

Computer axial tomography (CAT) scan – Machine that visualizes the inside of the human body using a combination of X-ray technology and computerized axial tomography; results are viewed on the computer.

Continuum of care – The philosophy that the health care system should facilitate an individual's care from complete independence to dependence.

Control research – Research whose major aim is to control symptoms, not cure the disease or condition. Pain medications control the symptoms of arthritis; they do not cure the underlying disease.

Coordination of benefits – If a service is covered under more than one policy, then the insurance companies determine which policy pays.

Copayment (coinsurance) – A payment made by the insured at the time services are received.

Core values – Values are shared attitudes and beliefs among group members. Core values are the central values of a culture.

Corporation – A legal form of business ownership that can have many owners. The percentage of the business owned is determined by the number of shares held by the owner, also known as a shareholder.

Cost/benefit analysis – The process of comparing the specific costs of a treatment to the benefits obtained by that treatment.

Cultural competence – The ability of health organizations and practitioners to recognize cultural beliefs, values, attitudes, traditions, language preferences, and health practices of specific cultural groups and to apply that knowledge to produce positive health outcomes.

Culture – An integrated and shared pattern of human behavior.

Curative medical care – Medical care that helps cure an already ill or infected person.

Curative research – Research whose major aim is to find a cure for a specific disease.

Current Procedural Terminology (CPT) – A part of the HCPCS used to code procedures and services performed by providers.

Deductible – An amount specified in the insurance policy that must be paid by the insured before the insurance company will pay.

Delivery models – Systems to bring a particular type of care to individuals and groups.

Demand – The amount of a good a buyer is willing to purchase at a given price.

Demographic – The data from human populations that describe vital statistics, size, and distribution.

Diagnostic tests – Tests ordered by a physician to provide information that assists in making a diagnosis.

Diploma program – Hospitals used to provide on-the-job training programs for nurses and award a diploma on completion. Very few diploma programs still exist.

Drug resistant – The term used to describe when a disease or bacteria are not affected or stopped by the use of common antibiotics and other drugs.

Eating disorders – A group of diseases that describes a patient's focus on food, obsessive eating, or not eating, along with faulty perception of body image.

Economic indicators – Key measurements that provide information about the health of the economy.

Electrocautery – The process of destroying tissue by an electrically heated instrument.

Electron beam computer tomography – Uses electron beams instead of X-rays for computerized axial tomography and also viewed on computer. Compared with the traditional CT scan, it does not require the patient to be completely still, is less enclosed, and costs more.

Employee Retirement Income Security Act of 1974 (ERISA) – Federal legislation that mandates how employer-funded benefit plans must be administered.

Enrollees – The employees who sign up for insurance coverage from the employer.

Enrollment period – The time period during which people, usually employees, can sign up for or change their insurance coverage.

Enteral nutrition – Nutrition delivered by a tube to the intestines. Example—nasogastric feeding tube.

Epidemic – A term used to describe a disease that is widespread in a population.

Epidemiology – The study of the nature, cause, control, and determinants of the frequency of disease, disability, and death in human populations. Also the study of the history of a disease and its distribution throughout a society (public health).

Ethnocentrism – The evaluation of behaviors according to one's own cultural beliefs.

Etiology – The study of the causes and origins of disease.

Exclusive Provider Organizations (EPOs) – Delivery networks in which patients must use the services of those providers.

Explanation of benefits (EOB) – A form sent to the patient that explains which claims were paid at what level.

Federal Employees Health Benefits Program (FEHBP) – An employer-sponsored health insurance program available to employees of the federal government.

Fee-for-service – A method of reimbursement that presets the fee that will be paid for the service provided.

For-profit – Making a profit is identified as the primary reason for the business to exist.

Foundation – A type of not-for-profit organization that raises money and then distributes it to other organizations in support of their programs.

Gatekeeping – A process of restricting access to services.

General and family practitioner – Physician who focuses on providing comprehensive health care to patients of all ages.

General hospitals – Hospitals that provide a range of services.

Generic drug – A drug sold or dispensed under a name that is not protected by a trademark, usually a chemical name or description (e.g., acetaminophen instead of Tylenol).

Gene sequencing – The process of determining the individual arrangement of nucleotides that compose a given gene; used extensively in drug research.

Gene therapy – The treatment of disease using normal or altered genes to replace or enhance nonfunctional or missing genes.

Governing board – A group who sets the overall direction for a group or business.

Gross Domestic Product (GDP) – The dollar value of all the final goods and services produced by businesses within a country's borders.

Group practice – A group of several physicians who practice as a group.

Healthcare Common Procedure Coding System (HCPCS) – A classification system used to code and process an insurance claim.

Health information record – Contains the patient's personal, financial, and social data as well as the medical data. The health information record replaces the term *medical record*.

Health Insurance Portability and Accountability Act of 1996 (HIPAA) – A federal law that mandates insurance portability and sets up procedures for electronic data exchange.

Health literacy – The degree to which individuals have the capacity to obtain, process, and understand basic information and services needed to make appropriate decisions about their health.

Health Maintenance Act of 1973 – Federal legislation that provided incentives for the formation of health maintenance organizations.

Health Maintenance Organization (HMO) – Employer prepays a flat fee to the HMO; employees receive services as they need them.

Health-related quality-of-life (HRQOL) – The physical and mental well-being of an individual that looks at the quality and quantity of a healthy life in terms of years.

Histology – The study of body tissues.

Hospitalists – Physicians who focus on providing care to hospitalized patients.

Human Genome Project – An international cooperative scientific project to map the 60,000 human genes that make up the human genetic code.

ICD-10-CM – The abbreviation for the *International Classification of Diseases, 10th Revision, Clinical Modification*. This classification is used to code office visits to process an insurance claim. ICD-10-CM became effective October 1, 2015, and replaced ICD-9-CM.

Imaging technology – A broad term referring to the many forms of technology that allow an image of the patient's body to be produced.

Implants – Medical devices that are placed inside the human body for therapeutic purposes, such as an insulin pump or artificial knee joint.

Indemnity – One party is exempted from incurred liabilities by the other party.

Independent practice association (IPA) model – The IPA markets the health plan. Physicians contract with the IPA to treat members of the HMO.

Infectious disease – A disease that can spread from person to person (versus a genetic disease or a disease that is not contagious).

Inflation – An increase in the price level.

Information technology – The business function that manages all the technology used to run the business and collects information for decision making.

Inpatient care – The patient needs care that requires being admitted to the hospital.

Institutional review board (IRB) – The group of people appointed by the government or a university to oversee any research on animals or humans.

Instrumental activities of daily living – Activities like managing money, telephoning, grocery shopping, personal shopping, using transportation, housekeeping, and managing medications.

Insured – The person who will receive benefits under the terms of an insurance policy.

Interest – The amount, stated as a percentage, paid to borrow money.

Internal medicine – An area of medicine that focuses on the body's organs, such as the heart, eyes, ears, kidneys, and the digestive, respiratory, and vascular systems.

Investigational new drug (IND) application – The notice to the FDA (Food and Drug Administration) that a company intends to begin clinical tests on humans.

Joint Commission (TJC) – National organization that evaluates and accredits health care organizations.

Kantian theory – An ethical theory developed by Immanuel Kant (1724–1804) that says a universal moral law obligates one to treat people as an end in itself.

Latex allergies – Many medical practitioners and patients are allergic to latex, which is the most commonly found material in gloves used in medical procedures.

Licensed practical nurse (LPN) – A nurse who has completed a state-approved program and passed a national exam. Generally, LPNs are supervised by RNs when providing patient care.

Limited liability partnership – A specific type of partnership arrangement in which a partner's liability is limited to the amount of the capital contribution.

Long-term care – The federal health care definition of long-term care is more than 60 days.

Magnetic resonance imaging (MRI) – Technology that uses electromagnetic radiation to visualize the body's soft tissues, such as the brain and spinal cord.

Major depression – A depression that lasts for a significant period of time or recurs frequently; a medical diagnosis.

Malpractice – The act of providing professional services that are below the standard of quality for that profession.

Managed care – Describes the combination of payments for health care and delivery of services into one system.

Management – The business function of planning, organizing, directing, and controlling the business's resources.

Market economy – An economy in which many sellers compete for customers.

Marketing – The business function that focuses on the exchange process between the business and its customers.

Medicaid – A federal and state program that funds health care primarily on the basis of the recipient's income.

Medical devices – The range of medical technologies that are used for therapeutic purposes, such as cardiac pacemakers and thermometers.

Medical history – The record of a patient's health, physicians' visits, symptoms, prescribed treatments, regular medications, and family medical history.

Medical imaging – Viewing the inside of the human body using a variety of techniques such as X-rays and CT scans.

Medical model – A viewpoint about health that focuses on the diagnosis and treatment of disease.

Medical nutrition therapy – The use of nutrition to support health in a patient.

Medical Power of Attorney – A person appointed by another who can give consent for medical care or can withhold medical care. It is a legal document that empowers the surrogate decision maker in all health care decisions if the patient is unable to make decisions.

Medical Practice Act – State legislation that sets out the requirements for physician licensure in that state.

Medical staff – Responsibility for quality patient care belongs to the physicians who make up the hospital's medical staff.

Medical technology – Therapeutic and diagnostic devices used to prevent, treat, diagnose, and assist patients medically. The X-ray machine is an example of medical technology.

Medicare – A federal program that pays health care costs for the elderly, the permanently disabled, and those with end-stage renal disease.

Medicare Advantage – A revision of the Medicare + Choice offered under Part C of Medicare.

Medicare Part A – This part of the Medicare program pays for inpatient hospital services, critical access to hospitals, and skilled nursing facilities.

Medicare Part B – This part of the Medicare program pays for physician services, outpatient hospital care, and some services and supplies.

Medicare Part C – This part of the Medicare program is an additional insurance plan intended to cover the gaps in Part A and Part B coverage.

Medicare Part D – This part of the Medicare program covers prescription drugs.

Medicare Prescription Drug, Improvement, and Modernization Act of 2003 – The most recent modification of the federal legislation. In particular, it added coverage for prescription drugs.

Mental health – The ability to cope with change, a positive outlook on life, ability to interact in close relationships in a loving and supportive manner, and the general feeling of well-being that can be assessed in the individual.

Minimally invasive surgery – Use of fiberoptics, guided images, microwave, and other technologies to do surgery rather than cutting large sections of tissue.

Monitoring – The regular review of disease data to determine changes in disease levels.

Monopoly – An economy with only one seller. The one seller is able to set whatever price it chooses.

Mood – The state of mind experienced at a particular time.

Mood disorder – An altered state of mind, such as the continuous sadness known as depression.

National codes (HCPCS level II codes) – The part of HCPCS used to code procedures and services not found in the CPT.

National Institutes for Health (NIH) – A group of federal governmental agencies responsible for the health of the nation.

Needlestick injuries – Health practitioners can be injured and exposed to disease if they are inadvertently stuck by a needle.

Network HMO – The HMO contracts with at least two group medical practices, described as "in network" to provide services.

New Drug Application (NDA) – The formal request to the FDA to be allowed to market a new drug.

Not-for-profit – The primary reason for the business to exist is some reason other than profit.

Not-for-profit hospitals – The primary purpose of the hospital is something other than profit.

Nurse Practice Act – State legislation that sets out the requirements for nurse licensure in the state.

Nurse practitioner (NP) – Advanced practice nurse who provides basic primary health care.

Nurse's aide – Health care worker who provides the most basic level of patient care, such as feeding and hygiene.

Nurse supervisor – A nursing position with more responsibilities and requiring more experience than a staff nurse.

Nursing home – An old-fashioned word designating a chronic care facility.

Nursing Interventions Classification (NIC) – A list of 554 interventions that are the nursing treatments of choice for each nursing diagnosis.

Nursing Outcomes Classification (NOC) – A list of 490 identified outcomes that are responsive to nursing care.

Nursing process – An organizing framework that provides a systematic method to deliver patient care.

Oligopoly – An economy with only a few sellers.

Osteopathic medicine – A process of treating patients by providing preventive and holistic care.

Outpatient care – Also referred to as ambulatory care. The patient does not require admittance to a hospital.

Outsourcing – The process of buying goods or services from another provider rather than performing them by the business.

Over-the-counter (OTC) – Drugs and medical devices that may be sold without a written health care provider's order. Aspirin and crutches are examples.

Parenteral nutrition – Any method of delivering nutrition that is not by mouth, such as by an intravenous line or by a direct tube into the stomach or intestine.

Parity – Equality; in this context, it means equality of benefits between insurance coverage for mental health and medical coverage.

Partnership – A legal form of business ownership that involves at least two people called *partners*.

Patient advocate – Hospital employee whose role is to take the side of the patient in all discussions and disputes.

Pediatrician – A physician who focuses on providing care to children.

Pharmaceuticals – Bioactive agents in the human body for therapeutic purposes (e.g., antibiotics).

Phlebotomist – A health care professional who collects blood samples.

Policy – The agreement, or contract, that describes all of the terms and conditions of an insurance policy.

Policy development – The process of making a collective decision about what needs to be done to protect the community's health.

Preauthorization – Many insurers require that certain procedures be authorized by the insurer before they are performed. Failure to obtain preauthorization may result in denial of the claim.

Predisposition – In medicine, a susceptibility to a disease or condition because of hereditary or other factors.

Preferred Provider Organization (PPO) – A delivery network that manages and negotiates contracts on behalf of the providers, who provide services at lower cost.

Premium – The price paid by the insured for insurance coverage.

Prepaid group practice model HMO – Physicians are employees of an independent group that contracts with the health plan to provide services.

Prepaid health plan (PHP) – Refers to types of health plans in which fixed payments are made before services are rendered.

Prescription drug – A drug that must have a health care provider's written order (prescription) to be dispensed.

Prevention efforts – Health programs and behaviors that prevent illness from occurring.

Preventive research – Research whose major aim is to find ways to prevent a disease or condition. For example, preventive research found that diet, exercise, and certain drugs like aspirin may prevent a second heart attack.

Primary care – Basic and routine care that can be delivered by a provider in an office or clinic.

Primary care physician – The physician who sees a patient regularly for routine and preventive care.

Privately owned hospitals – Hospitals owned by non-government entities.

Production – The business function that designs and manages the process that manufactures the business's products.

Profit – The amount left when a business subtracts its expenses from its revenues. If the amount is a negative number, it is a loss.

Proprietary – Owned by an individual or group of individuals: a for-profit arrangement.

Prospective payment system (PPS) – A payment system in which the amount of reimbursement is determined prior to the patient receiving services and is based on the patient's classification into a diagnostic-related group (DRG).

Public hospitals – Hospitals owned by the federal, state, or local government.

Quarantine – Forced isolation of a person to prevent a disease from spreading.

Radio frequency ablation (RFA) – Uses microwaves to destroy tissue.

Reciprocity agreement – An agreement between two states in which each accepts the professional licensing requirements of the other.

Recombination – The genetic process of new gene combinations that gives rise to offspring that have a combination of genes different from those of either parent.

Registered nurse (RN) – A nurse who develops and manages a nursing care plan for a patient.

Research and development (R&D) – The process of examining and bringing a product to market.

Residency – The last stage of physician training. After medical school, the student completes on-the-job training in his or her specialty.

Residential care – A living arrangement in which the person resides or lives full-time at a facility.

Rights theory – An ethical theory that believes people have certain basic rights as human beings and as citizens.

Risk factors – Anything that contributes to a person getting ill. A feature of someone's habits, genetic history, or personal history that increases the probability he or she will get a particular disease or injury. Smoking is a risk factor for lung cancer.

Risk of loss – The probability that the insured-against event will occur.

Risk pooling – The process of combining all the insureds into one group so the group's overall risk of loss is reduced.

Sandwich generation – The generation that is currently working and taking care of children and parents, thus sandwiched between two dependent age groups.

Secondary care – Usually involves routine hospitalization and surgery on a short-term basis.

Self-insured plan – A plan where an employer pays for employees' health care.

Self-referral arrangements – Health care providers are prohibited under federal law from referring patients to laboratories or other health services in which they have a financial interest.

Sick role – A pattern of behavior that is expected by the culture from a person who is defined as sick.

Single payer system – The financing of the costs of delivering universal health care for an entire population through a single insurance pool out of which costs are met.

Sole proprietorship – A legal form of business ownership that has only one owner.

Solo practice – A self-employed physician who practices alone.

Somatic – Affecting the body separate from the mind. For example, warm baths are a somatic treatment for calming the body.

Spend down – Redistributing assets so that the individual will be Medicaid eligible.

Staff model HMO – Physicians are employees of the HMO and paid a salary.

Staff nurse – An entry-level position for a nurse.

State Board of Nursing – Each state has an agency that oversees the profession and accredits educational programs.

Subculture – A group within a main culture that accepts the standards of the main culture, but has distinctive customs and values.

Supervised clinical experience – Nursing students obtain hands-on experience with patients as part of their education.

Surgeon – A physician who performs operations.

Surveillance – The continuous search for and documentation of disease in public health.

Sustainable competitive advantage – Anything about a business that allows it to outperform other businesses and maintain its position over time.

SWOT analysis – A method used by businesses to analyze the external environment.

Talk therapy – Psychotherapy invented by Sigmund Freud that involves primarily talking rather than somatic or drug therapy.

Technician – A person who performs the routine tasks in a laboratory setting.

Technologist – A professional who performs testing services. A technologist usually has more training than a technician.

Technology – The application of knowledge based on inventions, innovations, and discoveries in science.

Tertiary care – Complex and specialized care delivered in specific institutional settings, such as burn treatment.

Therapy – Remedial treatment of a disorder.

Third-party administrator (TPA) – A company that manages the paperwork for an employer who establishes a self-insured plan.

TRICARE – A health insurance program offered by the Department of Defense to military personnel.

Unemployment – A lack of jobs in an economy for those willing and able to work.

Usual, customary, and reasonable payment program (UCR) – A method of reimbursing providers by examining what other providers are paid for that service.

Utilitarianism – An ethical theory that believes resources should be distributed to achieve the maximum benefit.

Utilization measures – Measures that indicate whether an organization is being used to its full capacity.

Vector – An organism that transmits disease-causing microbes from infected individuals to other persons or from infected animals to human beings. Fleas were the vectors from rats to people in the great plagues.

Wellness model – A viewpoint about health that focuses on the prevention of disease.

Workers' compensation – A program that provides health care benefits to employees who are injured on the job.

Index